Atlas of Postmenopausal Osteoporosis
Third Edition

René Rizzoli
Division of Bone Diseases,
Department of Rehabilitation and Geriatrics
University Hospitals, Faculty of Medicine, Geneva, Switzerland

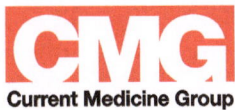
Current Medicine Group

Published by Current Medicine Group, 236 Gray's Inn Road, London, WC1X 8HL, UK

www.currentmedicinegroup.com

First published 2004
Second edition 2005
Third edition 2009

ISBN 978 1 85873 443 9

This publication has been made possible through an educational grant from Servier. Sponsorship of this copy does not imply the sponsor's agreement with the views expressed herein. Although every effort has been made to ensure that drug doses and other information are presented accurately in this publication, the ultimate responsibility rests with the prescribing physician. Neither the publisher nor the authors can be held responsible for errors or for any consequences arising from the use of the information contained herein. Any product mentioned in this publication should be used in accordance with the prescribing information prepared by the manufacturers. No claims or endorsements are made for any drug or compound at present under clinical investigation.

Commissioning editor: Ian Stoneham
Project editor: Lisa Langley
Designer: Joe Harvey and Taymoor Fouladi
Production: Marina Maher

Contents

Author biographies		v
Acknowledgements		viii
Introduction		ix
1	**Pathophysiology of postmenopausal osteoporosis**	**1**
	Bone anatomy and physiology	1
	Bone acquisition and peak bone mass	3
	Role of genetic factors	3
	Definition of osteoporosis	4
	The role of estrogen deficiency in the pathogenesis of osteoporosis	4
	The role of vitamin D and nutritional factors in postmenopausal osteoporosis	5
	References	31
2	**Epidemiology and diagnosis of postmenopausal osteoporosis**	**33**
	Prevalence of postmenopausal osteoporosis and the different fractures	33
	Risk factors	33
	Vertebral deformity and fracture	34
	Hip fracture	34
	Other types of fracture	34
	Diagnosis of osteoporosis	34
	Economic cost of fractures	37
	Effect of fractures on independence, quality of life, and mortality	37
	References	60
3	**Bone quality and strength**	**61**
	Determinants of bone strength	61
	Evaluation of bone strength	63
	References	82
4	**Prevention and treatment of postmenopausal osteoporosis**	**83**
	Goals of intervention	83
	Nonpharmacological approaches	83
	Pharmacological approaches	84
	Long-term management of postmenopausal osteoporiosis	93
	References	112
5	**Conclusion**	**115**
	Index	**117**

Author biographies

Editor

René Rizzoli is an internist and endocrinologist, with a subspecialty focus on metabolic bone diseases, osteoporosis and disorders of mineral metabolism. He is Professor of Medicine at the University Hospital of Geneva, Geneva, Switzerland and Head of the Division of Bone Diseases of the Department of Rehabilitation and Geriatrics. He is also chairman of this department. The Division of Bone Diseases is a World Health Organization (WHO) collaborating center for osteoporosis prevention. Professor Rizzoli is a member of the Executive Committee of the International Osteoporosis Foundation (IOF), and is the chairman of the Scientific Advisory Board of the European Society for Clinical and Economical Aspects of Osteoporosis and Osteoarthritis. He has also been chairman of the Committee of Scientific Advisors of the IOF, a position which he held for two mandates, and is a former president of the Swiss Association against Osteoporosis. He has chaired the scientific program committee of three consecutive IOF World Congresses on Osteoporosis. Professor Rizzoli is the Editor of the journal *Bone* and Associate Editor of *Osteoporosis International*, and has authored more than 550 articles and book chapters. He is involved in both basic and clinical research projects investigating hormone action, regulation of bone growth, mineral homeostasis, pathophysiology of osteoporosis and the role of nutrition, calcium, bisphosphonates, selective estrogen modulators (SERMs) and strontium ranelate in the prevention and treatment of osteoporosis.

Contributors

Patrick Ammann is an internist with a subspecialty focus on metabolic bone diseases, osteoporosis and disorders of mineral metabolism. He leads a preclinical investigation group on Osteoporosis and Bone Metabolism at the Division of Bone Diseases of the Geneva Department of Rehabilitation and Geriatrics, Geneva, Switzerland. The Division of Bone Diseases is a WHO collaborating center for osteoporosis prevention and bone diseases. Dr Ammann is involved in both basic and clinical research projects, investigating skeletal development, pathophysiology of osteoporosis, effect of nutrition and antiosteoporotic treatments (bisphosphonates, SERMs and strontium ranelate, parathyroid hormone, insulin-like growth factor and growth hormone) on bone mechanical properties and their determinants. He is also in charge of a rehabilitation unit for patients with osteoporotic fractures at the University Geriatric Hospital in Geneva. He has received numerous awards, both international and national, for his contribution to the understanding of metabolic bone disease pathophysiology.

Juliet Compston is Professor of Bone Disease and Honorary Consultant Physician at Cambridge University School of Clinical Medicine, Cambridge, UK. She obtained her medical degree at the Middlesex Hospital, London University, London, UK, with a distinction in Medicine. Professor Compston is actively involved in research into metabolic bone disease. Her research interests include the effects of glucocorticoids in bone and the role of megakaryocytes in bone remodelling. Recently her work has focused on secondary osteoporosis, particularly associated with liver transplantation and with cystic fibrosis. Professor Compston is a member of the board of the International Osteoporosis Foundation (IOF) and a board member of the International Bone and Mineral Society. She is Leader and Chair of the European Commission/IOF Call to Action for Osteoporosis, a Trustee of the Medical Board of the National Osteoporosis Society (NOS) and serves on the MHRA Expert Advisory Group on Women's Health. She is an Associate Editor of the *Journal of Bone and Mineral Research* and serves on the editorial board of *Bone* and *Osteoporosis International*. She is Chair of the

National Osteoporosis Guideline Group (NOGG) and a member of the Osteoporosis Guidelines Development Group for the National Institute of Clinical Excellence (NICE). She chaired the Guideline Development Group for the Royal College of Physicians Guidelines on the Prevention and Treatment of Glucocorticoid-induced Osteoporosis, and the Royal College of Physicians Working Group for the Update on Management of Postmenopausal Osteoporosis. She is Past President of the Bone and Tooth Society and the International Society of Bone Morphometry. In 2006 Professor Compston was awarded the National Osteoporosis Society's Kohn Foundation Award, which recognizes outstanding achievement in the field of osteoporosis. In 2009 she received the International Bone and Mineral Society John G. Haddad, Jr. Award, which recognizes outstanding contributions to clinical research in bone and mineral metabolism that have led to significant changes in understanding of physiology or disease, or to changes in disease management or prevention.

Serge Ferrari is Professor of Osteoporosis, Genetics and Medicine at the Geneva Faculty of Medicine, and Medical Associate at the Department of Rehabilitation and Geriatrics at the University Hospital of Geneva, Switzerland. He serves on the teaching committee of the Geneva Faculty of Medicine and teaches internal medicine, pathophysiology and bone metabolism to undergraduate students. After graduating from the Geneva University Faculty of Medicine in Switzerland (1989) he undertook a residency in internal medicine at the University Hospital of Geneva where he became Chief-Resident. From 1997–2001, he was a post-doctoral fellow at the Beth Israel Deaconess Medical Center in Boston, USA, during which time he was appointed Instructor in Medicine at Harvard Medical School (2000). Professor Ferrari has published more than 150 articles and book chapters in the bone field. He is a member of the editorial board of a number of journals, including *Journal of Bone and Mineral Research, Osteoporosis International* and *Bone*. He is also Editor-in-chief of *BoneKEy*, an on-line journal and knowledge environment of the International Bone & Mineral Society (IBMS). Professor Ferrari is president of the Swiss Bone and Mineral Society and a member of the council of scientific advisors of the International Osteoporosis Foundation (IOF). He is also a founding member and sits on the board of directors of the International Society of Nutrigenetics and Nutrigenomics (ISNN). He is the recipient of many international awards, as well as three-times winner of the clinical research award from the Swiss Bone and Mineral Society. Professor Ferrari's current research interests include bone growth and fragility in childhood, genetics of osteoporosis, and the molecular mechanisms of parathyroid activity and bone remodeling.

Harry K Genant is Professor Emeritus of the University of California San Francisco, California, USA, and a member of the Board of Directors of CCBR-SYNARC, Inc. He received his medical degree from Northwestern University in Chicago, Illinois, USA, and completed his internship on the Osler Service at Johns Hopkins University in Baltimore, Maryland, USA. In 1998 he co-founded Synarc, Inc, a global contract research organization specializing in the management of quantitative imaging and biomarkers in large, multicenter, multinational, pharmaceutical drug trials. He serves as a member of the Board and Senior Consultant for what is now CCBR-SYNARC, INC. Professor Genant has been editor or co-editor of more than 30 books and author or co-author of more than 170 chapters or invited articles, over 600 articles in peer-reviewed scientific and medical journals, and over 1500 abstracts presented at national and international scientific and professional gatherings. He is Associate Editor of *Bone* and a member of the editorial boards of *Osteoporosis International*, and the *Journal of Clinical Densitometry*. Among the numerous awards and honors Dr Genant has received are honorary lifetime memberships of the American Academy of Orthopaedic Surgeons and of the International Society for the Study of the Lumbar Spine. He is an honorary member of the Italian Radiolologic Society, the Chinese Osteoporosis Society, the Chilean Society of Osteology, the Hungarian Society of Osteology, and the European Society of Skeletal Radiology. He is a Fellow of the American College of Radiology and an Honorary Fellow of the Royal College of Radiologists. He was named Outstanding Physician of the Year by the International Society for Clinical Densitometry in 1998. Dr Genant has served as President of the Association of University Radiologists, President of the International Skeletal Society, Scientific Chair or President of the First through Sixth International Congresses on Osteoporosis in China, Co-Chair of the Second International Conference on Osteoporosis in Japan, Chair of the WHO Task Force on Osteoporosis, Chair of the International Steering Committee for Artificial Gravity for the joint US, German and Russia Space Programs, Member of the Radiologic Devices Panel of the US Food and Drug Administration, Member of the Board of Directors of the International Osteoporosis Foundation and Co-Director of the IOF Global Initiative on Vertebral Fracture Assessment and the IOF Bone Quality Working Group.

Audrey Neuprez is a research student at the University of Liège, Liège, Belgium, where she completed a Masters degree in Epidemiology, Public Health and Health Economics. Her research interests include the epidemiology of musculoskeletal disorders, with a particular interest in quality of life assessment. She is currently involved in the development of new tools to assess the cost-effectiveness of antiosteoarthritis medications with a particular emphasis on measuring health utility in patients with advanced stages of osteoarthritis, before and after hip and knee replacement surgery.

Jean-Yves Reginster is Professor of Epidemiology, Public Health and Health Economics and President of the Department of Public Health Sciences at the University of Liege, Belgium. He is also Head of the University Center for Investigation in Bone and Articular Cartilage Metabolism. Professor Reginster is a member of many national and international societies and is President of the Group for the Respect of Ethics and Excellence in Science (GREES) and the European Society for Clinical and Economic Aspects of Osteoporosis and Osteoarthritis (ESCEO). He has published some 600 original articles and over 60 book chapters. His interests revolve around bone-related pathologies, such as metabolic bone diseases, prevention and treatment of postmenopausal osteoporosis and osteoarthritis.

Johann D Ringe trained in medicine at the Universities of Göttingen (Germany), Montpellier (France) and Heidelberg (Germany). He is a Professor at the University of Hamburg and Cologne and is Head of the Department of General Internal Medicine (Rheumatology/Osteology) and of the West German Osteoporosis Center (WOC) at the Klinikum Leverkusen (University of Cologne), Cologne, Germany. He is a member of a number of national and international societies and has published over 500 articles, book chapters and books. He is on the editorial board and serves as a reviewer for a number of national and international journals. His research interests include the treatment of established osteoporosis with antiresorptive, osteoanabolic, or combined therapeutic strategies, preventive or therapeutic efficacy of calcium, vitamin D, alfacalcidol and SERMs in osteoporosis as well as the management of corticosteroid-induced osteoporosis and osteoporosis in men.

Acknowledgements

We would like to thank Professor Juliet Compston, Addenbrooke's Hospital, Cambridge, UK, for writing the Introduction to Chapter 1 and for providing additional material for, and reviewing, the complete text.

Introduction

René Rizzoli

Menopause is the time in a woman's life when reproductive capacity ends. Ovaries decrease their activity and the production of sex hormones ceases. This period may be associated with a large variety of symptoms affecting the cardiovascular and urogenital systems, as well as skin, hair and bone. Bone capital is accumulated by the end of the second decade and remains more or less constant up to the time of menopause. Sex hormone deficiency leads to accelerated bone turnover, a negative balance and microarchitectural deterioration, which compromises bone strength, thereby increasing bone fragility and, thus, fracture risk. By the age of 80, it is estimated that 50% of trabecular bone will have been lost.

Natural menopause occurs between the ages of 45 and 54 years all over the world. This age does not appear to have changed significantly over the centuries. In contrast, since the middle of the 19th century, life expectancy, particularly in women, has increased considerably, with most women living to the age of 80 years or more in many regions of the world. This means that at the age of 50 years, a woman will live for more than 30 years without bone protection by sex hormones. This represents more than one-third of a woman's life. At the age of 50 years, the lifetime risk to experience a fracture is about 50% (ie, one out of two women will have a fracture during this period).

In 2008, it was estimated that more than 700 million women were older than 50 in the world. This number should reach 1.2 billion by 2030. Osteoporotic fractures mainly include vertebrae, proximal femur, forearm and proximal humerus. The number of fractures of the proximal femur is expected to increase fourfold by 2030. In the book "Bone Formation and Repair", published in 1994, W.C. Hayes declared:

"If the prevalence of hip fracture continues to rise at current rates, it may well be that in the next few decades, orthopaedists will do little else but treat this problem".

This illustrates just how much osteoporosis threatens the health and quality of life of women with postmenopausal osteoporosis. This third edition of the atlas discusses the pathophysiology, epidemiology, diagnosis, prevention and treatment of postmenopausal osteoporosis, as well as the importance of bone quality and strength in fracture risk and osteoporosis therapy. It is hoped that it will be of interest and help for all professionals at the forefront of managing patients with osteoporosis.

Chapter 1

Pathophysiology of postmenopausal osteoporosis

Serge Ferrari and Johann D Ringe

Bone anatomy and physiology

The skeleton provides a rigid framework for the body, protecting vital organs, acting as a site for the attachment of muscles, and housing the bone marrow. It contains 99% of total body calcium, and plays a major role in the preservation of calcium and phosphate homeostasis, providing a reservoir from, or into, which these ions can be transported. Hence, in the absence of adequate amounts of calcium absorbed from the intestine, bone lysis will maintain serum calcium levels at the expense of bone strength.

Bone matrix and mineral

Bone is a highly specialized tissue consisting of an extracellular matrix within which bone mineral is deposited (Figure 1.1). Bone matrix is composed of type 1 collagen (Figure 1.2), proteoglycans, and a number of noncollagenous proteins, including osteopontin, osteocalcin, matrix Gla protein, thrombospondin, fibronectin, and bone sialoproteins. It is also a rich store of growth factors, including insulin-like growth factors (IGFs), transforming growth factor beta (TGF-β), fibroblast growth factors (FGFs), platelet-derived growth factors (PDGFs), and various bone morphogenetic proteins (BMPs). Bone mineral is composed predominantly of hydroxyapatite.

Bone macro- and microarchitecture

At the macroscopic level there are two types of bone: cortical (compact) and trabecular (cancellous) (Figure 1.3). Cortical bone comprises approximately 80% of the bone mineral mass of the whole skeleton, and is found in the shafts of long bones and outer surfaces of flat bones, whereas trabecular bone represents approximately 80% of the bone surfaces, and is found mainly at the ends (metaphysis and epiphysis) of long bones and inside flat bones and vertebrae. The mechanical strength of cortical bone increases with its diameter (or cross-sectional area) and thickness, decreases with cortical porosity (as seen during aging), whereas the strength of cancellous bone is mainly determined by the number and thickness of trabeculae and their horizontal connections [Seeman et al. 1997]. Trabecular bone is remodeled more rapidly and is therefore also more rapidly affected by conditions associated with increased bone turnover than cortical bone, as seen in early postmenopausal women.

Bone cells

There are three types of specialized bone cells, namely osteoclasts, osteoblasts, and osteocytes. Osteoclasts are bone-resorbing cells that are derived from hematopoietic cells of the monocyte/ macrophage lineage (Figure 1.4). Differentiated osteoclasts (Figure 1.5) are multi-nucleated cells with a ruffled membrane oriented to the surface of the bone which secrete the acid and enzymes (such as matrix metalloproteases, and cathepsin K) necessary for dissolution/digestion of the bone matrix [Rodan et al. 2008]. Osteoblasts are derived from pluripotent mesenchymal stem cells (MSCs), and their main function is the synthesis of the bone matrix (osteoid) and its subsequent mineralization (Figure 1.6). The latter requires two factors, type 1 collagen and alkaline phosphatase (ALP), which are markers of osteoblast activity [Murshed et al. 2005]. Osteocytes are terminally differentiated osteoblasts that have become embedded into the mineralized bone matrix (Figure 1.7). Whether or not they retain the ability to synthesize a mineralized bone matrix remains uncertain, however osteocytes constitute approximately 90% of bone cells in the adult skeleton. They are connected to one another and to osteoblastic cells on the bone surface by an extensive network of canaliculi, which contain the bone extracellular fluid. Osteocytes act as mechanosensors in bone, sensing physical strains and microdamage, and initiating the appropriate modeling and/or remodeling response [Bonewald, 2007].

Regulation of bone cells development and activity

The differentiation and activation of osteoblasts and osteoclasts is regulated by a few transcription factors (TFs) (Figure 1.8) and several local factors (mainly cytokines and growth factors [GFs]) produced by bone cells themselves and bone marrow/hematopoietic cells, as well as systemic factors/ hormones (Figure 1.9 and 1.10) [Cohen, 2006]. Experiments of nature and/or humans have delineated some of the factors that play an essential role in this processes, among which the TFs Runx2/ cbfa1 and Osx (osterix) are necessary for development of the osteoblastic lineage [Yang & Karsenty, 2002; Komori, 2006; Heino & Hentunen, 2008]. In contrast the TF Ppar gamma represses osteoblastogenesis and leads MSCs to become adipocytes, a phenomenon that may play an important role in the aging skeleton [Pei &Tontonoz,. 2004]. The LDL-receptor related protein 5 and/or 6 (Lrp5, Lrp6) with its co-receptor frizzled (Fzd), its agonists (Wnts) and antagonists (Dickkopf, Dkk1, and sclerostin, SOST), which signal through the canonical β-catenin pathway, is a major regulator of bone formation [Baron & Rawadi, 2007]. Although the specific factors that lead to terminal differentiation of osteoblasts into osteocytes remain unclear, the latter are characterized by the expression of a number of specific factors, including sclerostin (see above), fibroblast growth factor (FGF-23), periostin, dentin matrix acidic phosphoprotein (DMP-1) and other molecules involved in the regulation of phosphate homeostasis and matrix mineralization [Komori, 2006].

The development of osteoclasts depends on several TFs, (ie, PU.1 and AP-1 family members such as Fos), and the nuclear factor of activated T cell (NFATc1). Moreover, osteoclast development requires the macrophage colony-stimulating factor (M-CSF) and a specific cytokine, receptor activator of nuclear factor kappa B ligand (RANKL), that is produced by osteoblasts and T lymphocytes and which binds to its receptor (RANK), a member of the tumor necrosis growth factor (TNF) receptor superfamily. RANKL/RANK also plays a fundamental role in osteoclasts activation and survival. B lymphocytes and other cells also produce osteoprotegerin (OPG), which is an antagonist of RANKL and prevents osteoclastogenesis [Teitelbaum & Ross, 2003; Kearns et al. 2008]. Hence, OPG and RANKL play an essential role in the coupling of osteoblasts with osteoclasts and represent a novel target for the pharmacological inhibition of bone resorption [Bonewald, 2007]. In contrast, the coupling factors from osteoclasts to osteoblasts are less well characterized; these may include GFs released by osteoclasts themselves and/or from the bone matrix during resorption (see above), as well as ephrins and ephrin receptors expressed on the surface of osteoclasts and osteoblasts.

Bone modeling and remodeling

Bone modeling during growth ensures adaptation of bone size and shape, increasing the bone mineral mass until the peak bone mass of the adult skeleton is reached (Figure 1.11). It results from either bone formation or bone resorption. During growth for instance, an intense bone forming activity occurs on the outer bone surfaces (the periosteum) *de novo*, ie, without prior bone resorption [Rauch et al. 2006], whereas endosteal apposition is predominant in girls during puberty. Low levels of periosteal bone modeling may persist during adult life and aging, more so in men than women, to explain the continuous increase in cortical bone diameter seen for instance at the femur neck. Bone remodeling (or turnover) occurs throughout life at both endocortical and trabecular bone surfaces, as well as intracortically, to ensure adaptation of the skeleton to its functional needs, to repair microdamage and to maintain serum calcium homeostasis. This is a surface-based phenomenon that involves the removal of a quantum of bone by osteoclasts, followed by the deposition of new bone by osteoblasts, within the lacunae formed [Parfitt, 2002]. Osteoblasts produce an uncalcified bone matrix called the osteoid, which after a lag phase of approximately 10 days begins to mineralize. Under normal circumstances, resorption is always followed by formation (a relationship known as coupling), and the amounts of bone resorbed, or formed, within each remodeling unit are quantitatively similar (balance). Each bone remodeling cycle takes between four and six months to complete, most of this time being occupied by formation (Figure 1.12).

Approximately 10% of the skeleton is renewed by remodeling each year (ie, the entire skeleton is renewed every 10 years). In addition to overall bone remodeling occurring "randomly" on all bone surfaces, a targeted bone remodeling occurs to remove microdamage (ie, microcracks) which may be initiated by osteocytes following disruption of the canaliculae and osteocytes apoptosis [Seeman & Delmas, 2006].

Bone acquisition and peak bone mass

During childhood and adolescence bone mass increases several fold, reaching a peak by the end of the second decade of life (Figure 1.13). In girls, bone mass accumulation peaks between 12 and 13 years of age and declines rapidly after menarche (Figure 1.14), whereas in boys it peaks between 13 and 14 years of age and may be sustained for at least one more year than in girls, leading to an average 15% higher peak bone mass in males compared to females (Figure 1.15). Peak bone mass also differs according to ethnic origin, being greater in blacks for instance, but differences can be largely explained by differences in body size [Roy, 2005]. Estrogen is essential for the normal closure of the growth plates in both sexes. Girls with delayed menarchae are taller but display a lower bone mass and thinner cortices [Chevalley et al. 2008]. Hence, sex steroids play a major role in the attainment of peak bone mass, and are responsible for the sexual dimorphism of the skeleton, the male skeleton being characterized by greater bone size, with a larger diameter and greater cortical thickness in the long bones [Vanderschueren & Bouillon, 1995]. Nevertheless, volumetric bone mineral density (BMD) at peak bone mass is similar in young adult men and women. Peak bone mass is determined by a number of factors, including genetics, physical activity (Figure 1.16), hormonal status, calcium intake (Figure 1.17), and more general aspects of nutrition. A 10% increase in peak bone mass may be equivalent to delaying the risk of postmenopausal osteoporosis by 5–10 years.

Role of genetic factors

Genetic factors are perhaps the most important determinants of peak bone mass, and may also influence age-related bone loss (Figures 1.18–1.19). Family history, particularly of a fragility (hip) fracture, is an important risk factor for osteoporosis, indicating the influence of heredity on BMD and other related determinants of bone fragility [Seeman et al. 1989; Torgerson, 1996; Kanis et al. 2008]. Twin and family studies have shown that genetic factors account for 50–85% of the variance in BMD, bone size and hip geometry [Ralston, 2002], and may also contribute 40–60% of the variance in bone turnover and microarchitecture. Additive genetic effects on fractures appear to be "only" 25–50%, pertaining to the additional influence of falls and the environment. Various single-gene mutations have been identified to cause bone fragility, including the well-known collagen type 1 alpha 1 (*COL1A1*) and alpha 2 (*COL1A2*) gene defects responsible for osteogenesis imperfecta. Inactivating mutations of the low-density lipoprotein receptor-related protein-5 (*LRP-5*) gene cause the osteoporosis/pseudoglioma syndrome, while activating mutations cause a variety of syndromes characterized by high bone mass and/or sclerosing bone dysplasias with increased bone strength [McGuigan, 2003; Ferrari et al. 2005]. Susceptibility to idiopathic osteoporosis and fractures, however, is not determined by single-gene mutations but by multiple common variations in the DNA sequence (ie, by gene polymorphisms). Single nucleotide polymorphisms (SNPs) occur at a frequency of 1 per 500–1000 base pairs in the human genome and rarely alter protein level and/or function. Nevertheless, numerous studies and meta-analyses of SNPs in osteoporosis candidate genes, such as *COL1AI*, estrogen receptor alpha (ERα) (eg, estrogen receptor 1 [*ESR1*]), vitamin D receptor (*VDR*), *LRP5*, interleukin-6 *(IL-6)*, bone morphogenetic protein 2 *(BMP-2)* and others, have shown association with BMD and/or fracture risk [Ferrari, 2008; van Meurs et al. 2008]. More recent hypothesis-free approaches investigating at once hundreds of thousands of SNPs across the whole genome (genome-wide association studies) have confirmed some of the above associations and started to identify additional polymorphisms associated with osteoporosis, including in the RANKL and OPG genes (*TNSF11*, *TNFRSF11b*). The sexual dimorphism of skeletal traits and osteoporosis risk may reflect differences in the expression of gene polymorphisms in the respective hormonal milieu of men and women [Karasik et al. 2008].

Definition of osteoporosis

Osteoporosis is defined as a reduction in bone mineral mass and bone quality, that is a disruption of bone microarchitecture and weakening of material properties (Figure 1.20), resulting in increased bone fragility, and increased fracture risk [Consensus Development Conference, 1993; NIH Consensus Development Panel on Osteoporosis Prevention, Diagnosis, and Therapy, 2001]. Thinning and increased porosity of the cortices are seen, together with conversion of trabecular plates into thinner rod-like structures and a decrease of trabecular number (Figure 1.21); furthermore, resorption areas in trabeculae represent stress risers that concentrate breaking forces and may ultimately lead to perforation of trabeculae resulting in reduced connectivity and failure of the trabecular bone structure [Seeman et al. 2006]. These changes, which are seen in postmenopausal osteoporosis and aging men and women, result from the combination of increased osteoclastic activity, and insufficient osteoblast function (ie, an increased and imbalanced bone remodeling activity that characterize this condition).

The role of estrogen deficiency in the pathogenesis of osteoporosis

Normal premenopausal levels of estradiol protect the skeleton against an increasing bone turnover with a negative bone balance. Accordingly early menopause is a major risk factor for postmenopausal osteoporosis (Figure 1.22). Estrogen deficiency is the major cause of postmenopausal bone loss in women, and decreases in biologically available estrogen levels also contribute to age-related bone loss in men [Riggs et al.1998]. In postmenopausal women the rate of this bone loss has been shown to be significantly associated with fracture risk [Sornay-Rendu et al. 2005]. After its onset, age-related bone loss continues throughout life in both men and women.

Skeletal effects of estrogen

In women, the large decrease in estrogen production associated with the menopause is responsible for increased bone turnover and continuous bone loss (Figures 1.23–1.24), and estrogen replacement at the menopause abrogates these changes [Christiansen et al. 1980; Lindsay et al. 1976]. Biochemical markers of bone resorption and formation can be measured in the blood and urine (Figures 1.25–1.26). Resorption markers include deoxypyridinoline (measured in urine) and amino and carboxy-terminal cross-linked telopeptides of type 1 collagen (NTX and CTX; measured in serum or urine). Serum levels of osteocalcin, bonespecific alkaline phosphatase, and amino-terminal propeptide of type 1 collagen (PINP), are examples of commonly used formation markers [Seibel & Woitge, 1999]. At the menopause, these markers of both resorption and formation increase, but can be restored to premenopausal values by estrogen replacement [Delmas et al. 2000]. Estrogen deficiency also plays a role in bone loss in older postmenopausal women (Figures 1.27–1.28), since estrogen replacement is effective in preventing bone loss in this age group [Quigley et al. 1987]. The mechanisms by which estrogen exerts its skeletal effects remain to be clearly defined. Many of its actions on bone are mediated via ERα, while the contribution of ERβ remains poorly characterized. Estrogen promotes osteoclast apoptosis [Nakamura et al. 2007; Khosla, 2007] while exerting an opposite effect on osteoblasts and osteocytes, preventing their death and enhancing their functions, including mechanotransduction in response to loading [Lee et al. 2003]. Estrogen deficiency is associated with the increased production of proresorptive cytokines by bone cells and cells in the bone marrow, including megacaryocytes and T cells [Weitzmann et al. 2005]. Factors involved include IL-1, -6 and -11, and TNFα, RANKL, and granulocyte-macrophage colony- stimulating factor (GM-CSF) [Compston, 2001; Eghbali-Fatourechi et al. 2003].

Other systemic factors implicated in bone turnover

Parathyroid hormone (PTH) also plays a major role in the regulation of bone turnover, both primary and secondary hyperparathyroidism being associated with osteopenia/osteoporosis. PTH increases bone turnover through the production of local factors, including IGF-1, PTH-related protein (PTHrP) and RANKL; by inhibiting the expression of sclerostin; and potentially by a cross-talk with the wnt/LRP5/6 signaling pathway [Goltzman et al. 2008]. Growth hormone (GH), acting both directly on bone and through the systemic production of IGF-1, is another important stimulus for both bone formation and resorption. Low levels of IGF-1 and/or GH are involved in the pathogenesis of osteoporosis associated low dietary protein intake [Rizzoli et al. 2001] and with anorexia nervosa, the latter also involving low levels of gonadal steroids. Bone metabolism is also linked to fat and energy metabolism through leptin and other adipokines, neuropetide Y (NPY), and the β-adrenergic system [Hamrick & Ferrari, 2008; Bonnet et al. 2008]. Eventually serotonin may exert inhibitory functions on osteoblasts and explain some of the Wnt/LRP5 effects as well as the negative influence of depression and serotonin-uptake inhibitors on the skeleton [Yadav. et al. 2008].

Skeletal effects of glucocorticoids

Glucocorticoids (GC) have complex effects on bone remodeling, and their use can lead to a rapid and early bone loss, osteoporosis and increased fracture incidence in the early stages of GC therapy (Figure 1.29). The predominant effect is reduction in bone formation, owing to reduced generation of osteoblast precursors, and increased apoptosis of osteoblasts and osteocytes. These effects are mediated both systemically, through a reduction in the level of GH/IGF-1 and sex steroids, and directly on bone cells [Canalis et al. 2007]. Accordingly, GC therapy is characterized by a rapid and sustained suppression of serum osteocalcin levels. In addition, particularly in the early phases of glucocorticoid therapy, there is evidence for increased osteoclastogenesis and reduced osteoclast apoptosis, resulting in increased bone resorption [Manolagas, 2000]. Again these effects result from both a decreased intestinal absorption of calcium by GC with secondary hyperparathyroidism, and from direct GC effects on bone cells leading to an increased production of RANKL, respectively reduced expression of OPG [Hofbauer et al. 1999].

The role of vitamin D and nutritional factors in postmenopausal osteoporosis

Although estrogen deficiency is strongly implicated in the pathogenesis of postmenopausal osteoporosis, nutritional factors also play an important role (Figure 1.30). Vitamin D insufficiency defined as serum 25-hydroxyvitamin D [25(OH)D] levels below 30 ng/ml (75 nmol/L) and resulting from poor sun exposure and/or skin synthesis, is commonly found in all populations, affecting up to 60–90% of older postmenopausal women [Lips et al. 2006]. Levels of 25(OH)D which fall below 20–30 ng/ml often result in secondary hyperparathyroidism, which can be aggravated with additional low calcium intake (<800 mg/day), favoring especially cortical bone loss [Steingrimsdottir et al. 2005]. Insufficiency of calcium (Figure 1.31), vitamin D, and protein (Figure 1.32) [Rizzoli & Bonjour, 2004] are particularly important in the pathogenesis of hip fractures [Rizzoli et al. 2001], and there is evidence that vitamin D supplementation of 800 IU/day (Figure 1.33) may reduce the risk of falls and the incidence of hip and other nonvertebral fractures by 20–30% [Chapuy et al. 1992; Bischoff–Ferrari et al. 2005]. Protein supplementation in undernourished, frail elderly may also contribute to improve bone mass and muscle function, particularly in the catabolic state following a hip fracture [Schurch et al. 1998].

Bone composition

Figure 1.1. Bone is composed of an organic and inorganic phase, of which approximately 70% by weight is mineral or inorganic matter, 5–8% is water, and the remainder is organic, or extracellular matrix. Of the inorganic matter, 95% is composed of calcium hydroxyapatite, and the remainder is impurities. Of the organic phase, 85% is composed of type I collagen (see Figure 1.2), and the remaining 15% is composed of small amounts of other collagens, several noncollagenous proteins, glycoproteins, and approximately 2% is made up of cells. Some of these noncollagenous proteins, such as osteocalcin, are specific to bone, while others, such as osteopontin, fibronectin, and various peptide growth factors, are also found in other connective tissues. The noncollagenous bone proteins are involved in the attachment of bone cells to bone matrix, and in regulating bone cell activity during the process of bone remodeling.

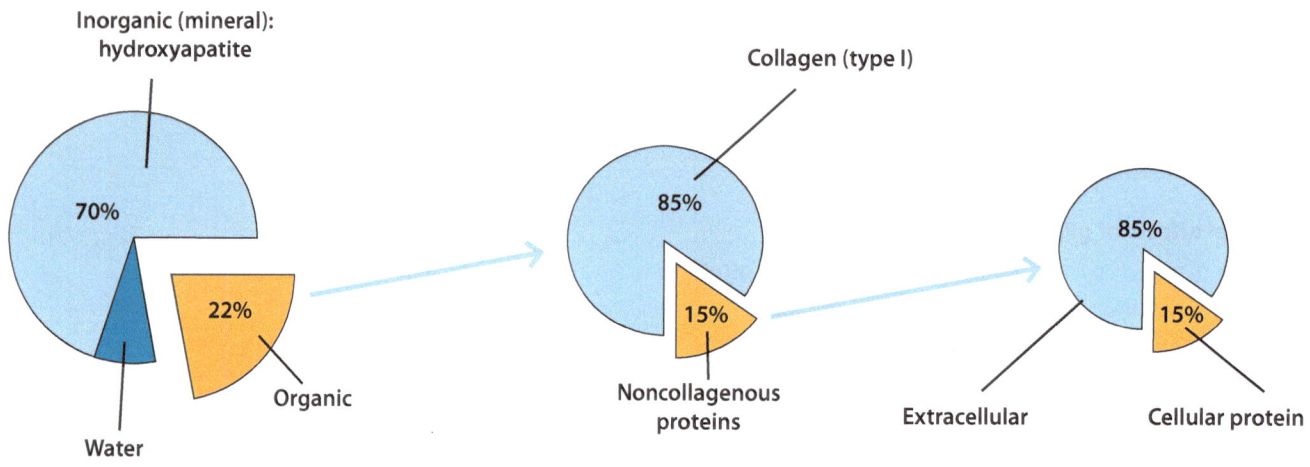

Bone collagen

Figure 1.2. The bone matrix is mainly formed of type 1 collagen, a fibrillar protein formed from three protein chains wound together in a triple helix, and produced in organized, parallel lamellae, which become cross-linked by specialized covalent bonds (pyridinium links) giving bone its strength. Type I collagen is laid down along with other collagenous proteins, noncollagenous proteins, glycoproteins, and small amounts of other proteins (absorbed from extracellular fluid) during bone formation by osteoblasts, creating the uncalcified bone matrix (osteoid). After a lag phase of approximately 10 days, the matrix becomes mineralized, as hydroxyapatite crystals are deposited in the spaces between collagen fibrils. **(a)** The scanning electron image shows bone collagen fibrils in both longitudinal and cross sections. **(b)** A back-scattered electron image of the regular patterns of collagen in layers in normal, or lamellar, bone.

(a)   **(b)**

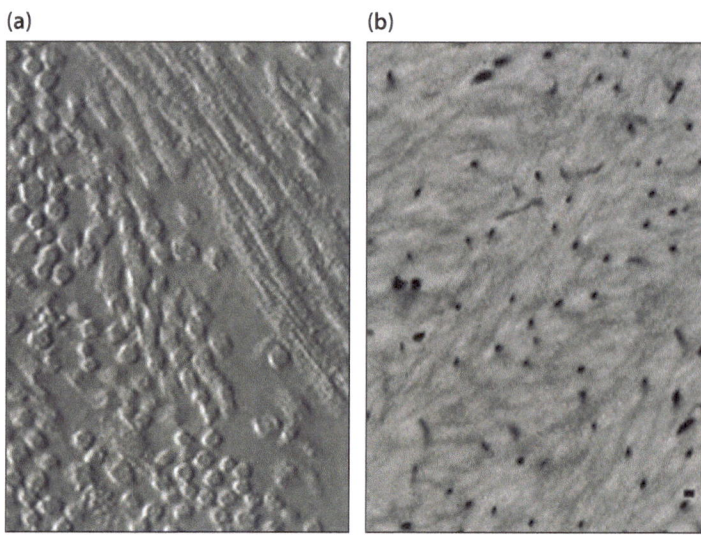

Cortical and trabecular bone

Figure 1.3. The normal human skeleton contains two types of bone: cortical (compact) bone, which is present in the shafts (diaphyses) of the long bones (eg, femur and tibia), and trabecular (spongy or cancellous) bone, which makes up most of the vertebral bodies and the ends of the long bones, (ie, the metaphysis and epiphysis). Cortical bone consists of compact bone arranged concentrically around central canals (the Haversian system) containing blood and lymphatic vessels, nerves, and connective tissue. Trabecular bone is composed of interconnecting plates within which lies the bone marrow. Adapted with permission from Standring S (Ed) Gray's anatomy – the anatomical basis of clinical practice, 39th edition. Edinburgh: Elsevier, 2004. Micro-CT image courtesy of R Mueller.

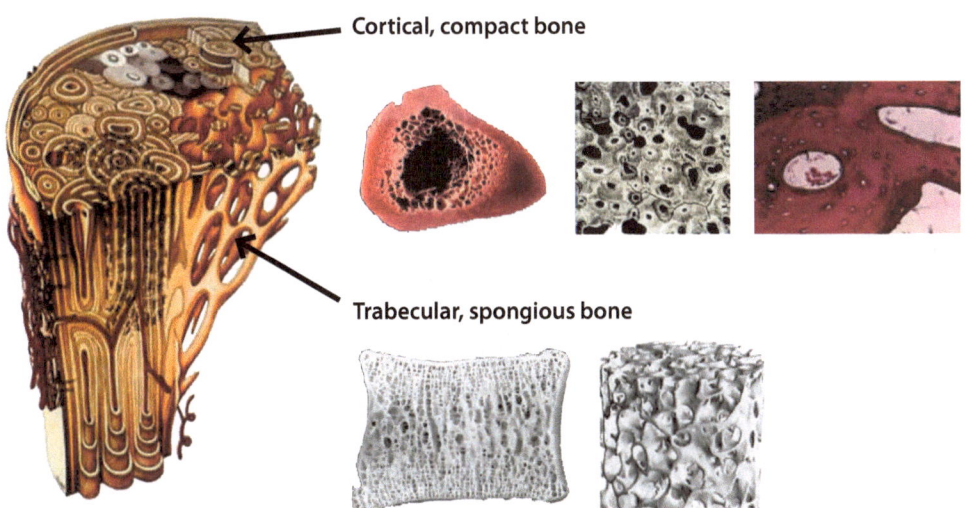

Cross-section of an activated osteoclast

Figure 1.4. Osteoclasts, which are multinucleated phagocytes, are rich in the enzyme tartrate-resistant acid phosphatase (TRAP). During the bone resorption process, mature osteoclasts form a tight seal over the bone surface, and resorb bone by secreting hydrochloric acid and proteolytic enzymes onto the bone surface. The acid dissolves hydroxyapatite, and this allows the proteolytic enzymes access to degrade collagen, and other bone matrix proteins. Important molecules in this phase include: carbonic anhydrase-II (CAII), which is necessary for acid generation; a subunit of the osteoclast proton pump encoded by the gene TCIRG1; cathepsin K, a proteolytic enzyme that is necessary for matrix degradation; and other matrix metalloproteases (MMPs). After resorption is completed, osteoclasts undergo apoptosis in the reversal phase, which heralds the start of bone formation.

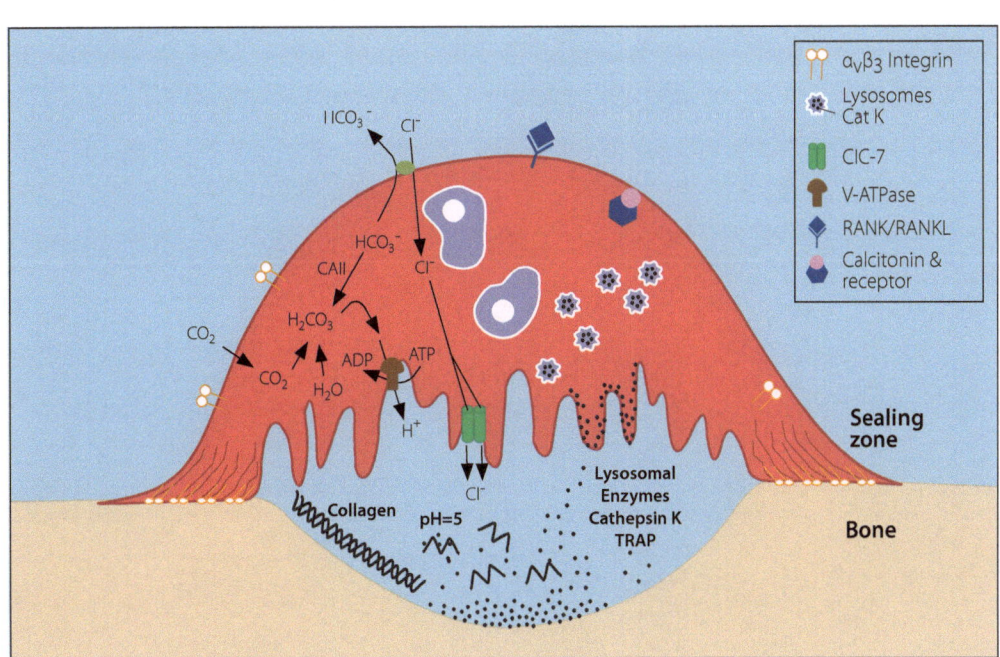

Differentiation of osteoclasts

Figure 1.5. Several transcription factors (such as PU.1 and Ffos), systemic and local factors (mainly cytokines, see Figure 1.9) are implicated in the regulation of osteoclast differentiation. However two factors are sufficient and necessary for the differentiation of early osteoclast precursors from hemopoietic stem cells (colony forming unit-monocyte/macrophage, CFU-M): macrophage colony-stimulating factor (M-CSF) and receptor activator of nuclear factor kappa B ligand (RANKL) binding to its receptor RANK. RANKL/RANK also influence the later stages of osteoclastogenesis by promoting differentiation of committed precursors to mature osteoclasts, stimulating bone resorptive activity of mature osteoclasts, and survival. RANKL is produced by osteoblasts and inflammatory cells , ie, dentritic cells (DC) and T lymphocytes. The latter may also play a role in activating bone resorption following estrogen deficiency. Osteoprotegerin (OPG), which is expressed by osteoblasts, bone marrow stromal cells, B lymphocytes and other cell types, inhibits osteoclast formation and activity by binding to the RANKL molecule and preventing it from activating RANK. Adapted from Boyle WJ, Simonet WS, Lacey DL. Osteoclast differentiation and activation. Nature 2003; 423:337–42.

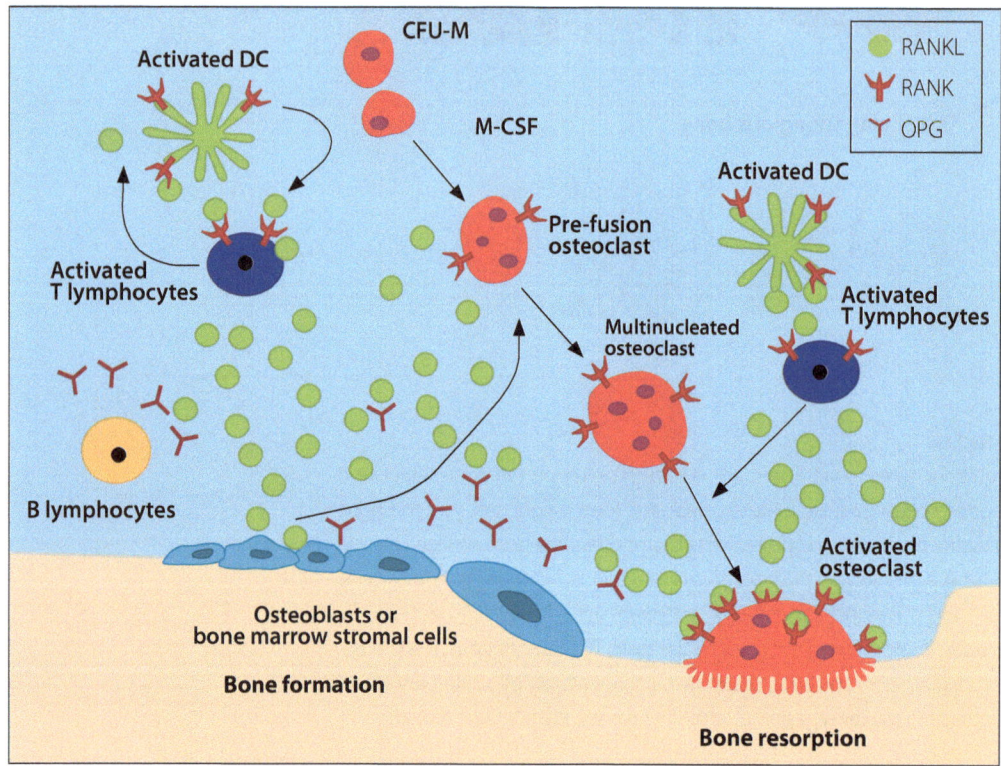

Stimulation of bone formation by osteoblasts

Figure 1.6. The Wnt-LRP5/6-β-catenin canonical signaling pathway plays a major, likely essential, role for the stimulation of bone formation by osteoblasts. **(a)** Following Wnt binding to its LRP5/6 and frizzled (Fz) co-receptors, the beta-catenin inhibitory complex containing glycogen synthase kinase (GSK)-3β is inactivated. β-catenin is then stabilized and accumulates in the cytoplasm. β-catenin consequently translocates into the nucleus where it affects gene expression. **(b)** This system has multiple extracellular antagonists, such as secreted Dickkopf (Dkk) proteins, that bridge LRP5/6 and the transmembrane protein Kremen, leading to inactivation of the receptors by internalization. Sclerostin (SOST), which is produced by osteocytes, also inhibits Wnt signaling through binding to LRP5/6. (a) and (b) reproduced with permission from Baron R, Rawadi G. Targeting the Wnt/beta-catenin pathway to regulate bone formation in the adult skeleton. Endocrinology 2007; 148:2635–43. **(c)** In transgenic mice overexpressing Dickkopf related protein 1 (Dkk1++), bone mineral density and trabecular bone structure are markedly reduced when compared with controls. Reproduced with permission from Li J, Sarosi I, Cattley et al. Dkk1-mediated inhibition of Wnt signaling in bone results in osteopenia. Bone 2006; 39:754–66. **(d)** In SOST-deficient mice, bone mineral mass and structure are markedly increased, as shown here by a dramatic thickening of the cortex. Reproduced with permission from Li X, Ominsky MS, Niu QT et al. Targeted deletion of the sclerostin gene in mice results in increased bone formation and bone strength. J Bone Miner Res 2008; 23:860–9.

(a)

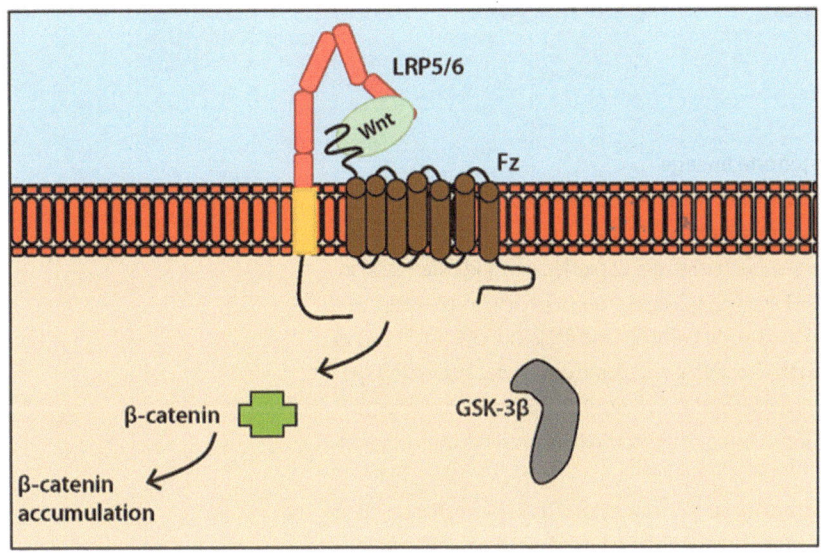

(c)

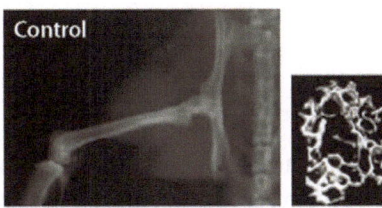
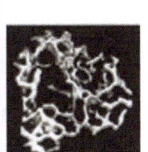
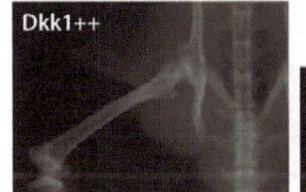
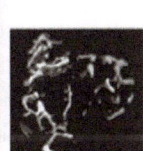

(b)

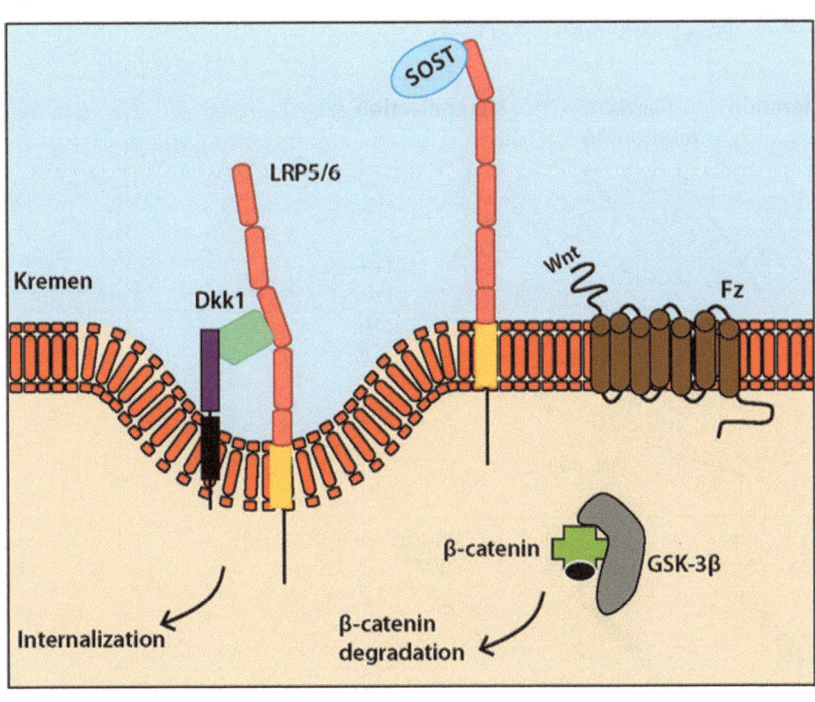

(d) Male

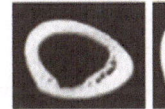
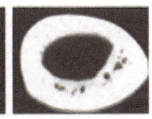

Control   SOST-deficient

Female

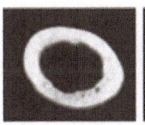
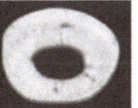

Control   SOST-deficient

Osteocytes

Figure 1.7. Osteocytes embedded in the bone matrix form a dense cellular network. During normal loading or ambulation, osteocytes send inhibitory signals to osteoclasts to maintain bone mass, while viable osteocytes are necessary to send signals activating osteoclasts in response to unloading. Osteocytes do not play a role in bone restoration in response to reloading after loss due to unloading. In the absence of load, the osteocyte sends signals to the osteoclast to resorb bone. But if the osteocytes are killed by diphtheria toxin (DT) injection and then reloaded, bone is nonetheless regenerated. These results indicate that the mechanisms responsible for maintaining bone mass with normal load are not the same as those for recovering bone mass after unloading.

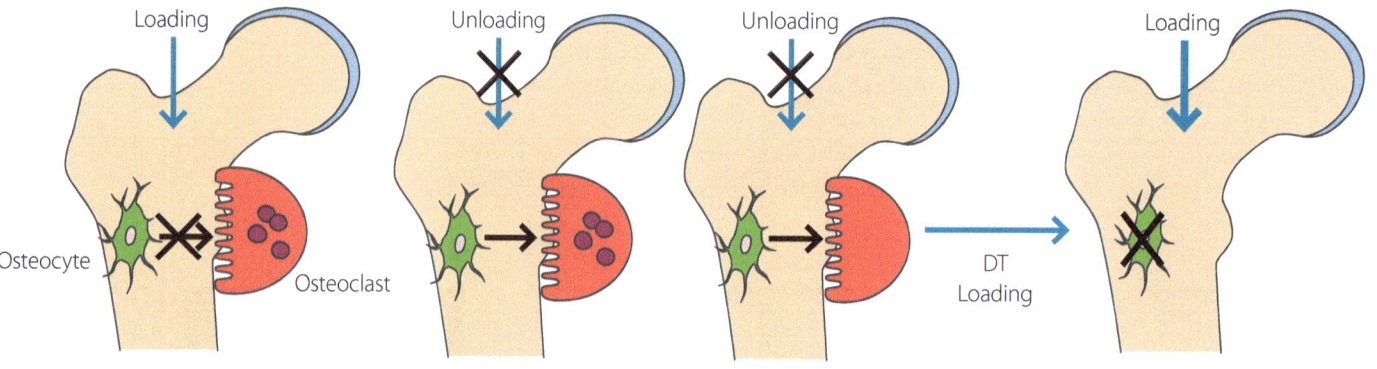

Activation of transcription factors in the osteoblast/osteocyte lineage

Figure 1.8. Commitment of pluripotent mesenchymal stem cells (MSCs) to the osteoblast/osteocyte lineage requires the sequential activation of transcription factors (TFs) Cbfa1/Runx2 and osterix (Osx). Additional TFs are also involved in osteoblast differentiation, such as ATF4 and Sox4. During the sequential stages of proliferation and differentiation, osteoblasts express specific genes including collagen 1 (COL1A1 and COL1A2 chains) and alkaline phosphatase (ALP), which are sufficient and necessary for matrix mineralization, bone sialoprotein (BSP), and finally osteocalcin (BGP) and osteopontin (OPN). Osteoblasts which become embedded in the bone matrix become osteocytes, expressing specific molecules implicated in matrix mineralization and phosphate homeostasis (DMP-1, FGF-23), as well as sclerostin (SOST), a major inhibitor of bone formation (see Figure 1.6). MSCs have the potential to differentiate into alternative cell types depending on the activation of specific TFs, such as peroxisome proliferation activated receptor gamma (PPARγ) for adipocytes, Sox9 for chondrocytes, and myogenic differentiation (Myod) for myocytes. ATF, activating transcription factor; Cbfa1, core binding factor alpha 1; c-Fos, cellular proto-oncogene; DMP, dentin matrix acidic phosphoprotein; FGF, fibroblast growth factor; MEPE, matrix extracellular phosphoglycoprotein; Sox, sex determining region Y high mobility group box. Adapted from Ferrari S. Cellular and molecular mechanisms of osteoporosis. In: Innovation in skeletal medicine. Edited by JY Reginster and R Rizzoli. Issy-Les-Moulineaux: Elsevier Masson, 2008; 19–46.

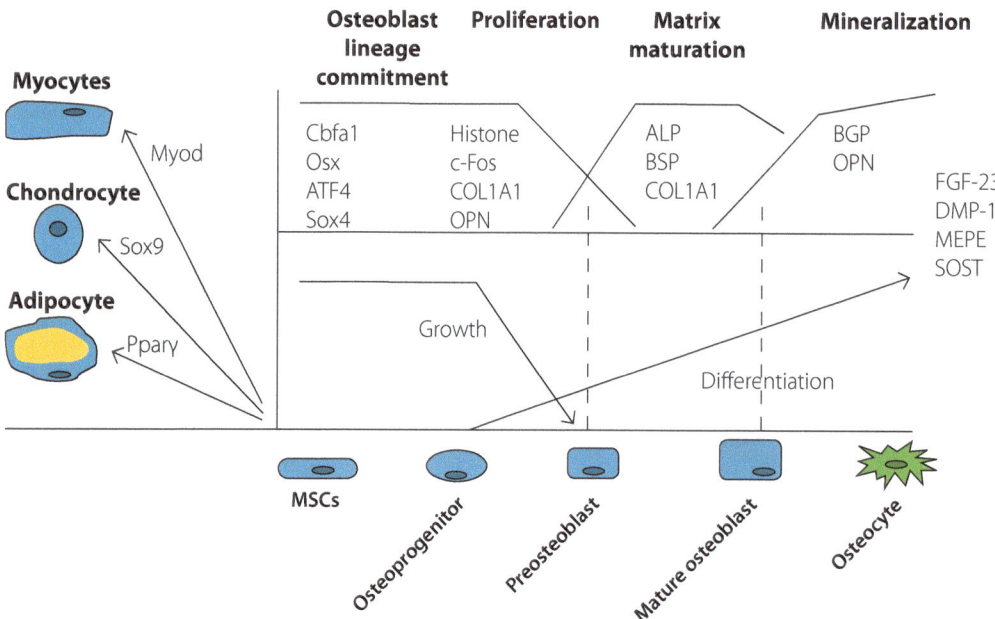

Factors influencing bone formation and resorption

Figure 1.9. The main stimulators and inhibitors of bone remodeling are shown in this figure. **(a)** Bone formation. **(b)** Bone resorption. Mechanical stimuli, and areas of microdamage, are likely to be important in determining the sites at which remodeling occurs in the normal skeleton. Increased bone remodeling may result from the local, or systemic, release of inflammatory cytokines, such as interleukin-1 (IL-1), and tumor necrosis factor (TNF) in inflammatory diseases. Several cytokines have a dual effect on the stimulation of bone resorption together with an inhibition of formation. Calciotropic hormones, such as parathyroid hormone (PTH) and 1,25-dihydroxyvitamin D, act together to increase bone remodeling on a systemic basis, allowing skeletal calcium to be mobilized for maintenance of plasma calcium homeostasis. Bone remodeling is also increased by other hormones, such as thyroid hormone, and growth hormone (GH), but is suppressed by estrogens, androgens, and calcitonin. Adipokines, such as leptin, and the adrenergic system are increasingly recognized as modulators of bone remodeling through the central nervous system (see Figure 1.10). CSF, colony stimulating factor; RANKL, receptor activator of nuclear factor kappa B ligand.

(a) Bone formation

Stimulators		Inhibitors
• PTH • PTH-related protein • Sex-steroids (E2 and T) • GH: insulin-like growth factor-1 • Thyroid hormone • Leptin (peripheral)	Systemic	• Glucocorticoids • Leptin (central nervous system) • B$_2$ adrenergic • Serotonin
• Mechanical stress • Transforming growth factor-β • BMPs (BMP-2) • Platelet-derived growth factors • Endothelial growth factor • Vascular endothelial growth factor • Insulin-like growth factors (IGF-1) • Fibroblast growth factors (FGF-2) • Prostaglandins • Wnt-LRP5/LRP6	Local	• Sclerostin • Noggin • Interleukin-1β, 7 • Interferon-γ • Tumor necrosis factor-α • Dickkopfs

(b) Bone resorption

Stimulators		Inhibitors
• PTH • PTH-related protein • 1,25(OH$_2$)D$_3$ • Thyroid hormone • B$_2$ adrenergic	Systemic	• Calcitonin • Sex-steroids (E2)
• RANKL • Macrophage-CSF • Granulocyte macrophage-CSF • Interleukin-1, 6, 7, 11, 15,17 • Interferon-γ • Tumor necrosis factor-α • Fibroblast growth factors • Prostaglandins	Local	• Osteoprotegerin • Transforming growth factor-β • Interferon-γ • Interleukin-4, IL-10, IL-13, IL-18 • Interleukin-1 receptor agonist

Bone turnover and bone mass

Figure 1.10. Bone turnover and bone mass are regulated by a number of systemic factors in response to changes in pubertal maturation and growth, body composition (including fat), dietary intake, and for the purpose of serum calcium and phosphate homeostasis. This figure provides an integrated view of the main hormonal influences on the skeleton (+, increases trabecular and/or cortical bone mass, - decreases bone mass). The central nervous system (CNS) is directly implicated through the release of growth hormone (GH) triggering the production of insulin-like growth factor-1 (IGF-1) by the liver, which stimulates bone formation, particularly at periosteal surfaces, while GH itself also has direct effects on bone remodeling. The CNS also mediates some of the effects of the adipocytic hormone leptin, which inhibits trabecular bone formation and stimulates resorption through a beta-2 adrenergic receptors relay, resulting in lower cancellous bone volume. In contrast, leptin and beta-1 adrenergic signaling may stimulate bone formation and directly increase cortical bone mass. Estradiol (E2) produced by the ovaries and through the conversion of androgens by aromatase (as found abundantly in fat), plays a fundamental role in the acquisition of bone mass in both genders and inhibits trabecular and endocortical bone remodeling thereafter, but might also exert a negative influence periosteal growth, while testosterone (T) promotes bone formation at this level. Parathyroid hormone (PTH) levels are regulated by the calcium sensing receptor (CaSR) on parathyroid glands as well as by circulating levels of $1,25(OH_2)D_3$. PTH is a main stimulus for bone remodeling and its physiological role is primarily to maintain serum calcium homeostasis. However, PTH is also a main stimulus for osteoblast differentiation and survival. Hence, PTH may either decrease or increase bone mass (+/-), depending on the mode and duration of the exposure. Eventually, the active form of vitamin D, $1,25(OH_2)D_3$ (calcitriol), is essential for bone mineralization through intestinal calcium absorption, but also directly stimulates bone turnover. ADRb1, adrenergic receptor β_1; ADRb2, adrenergic receptor β_2.

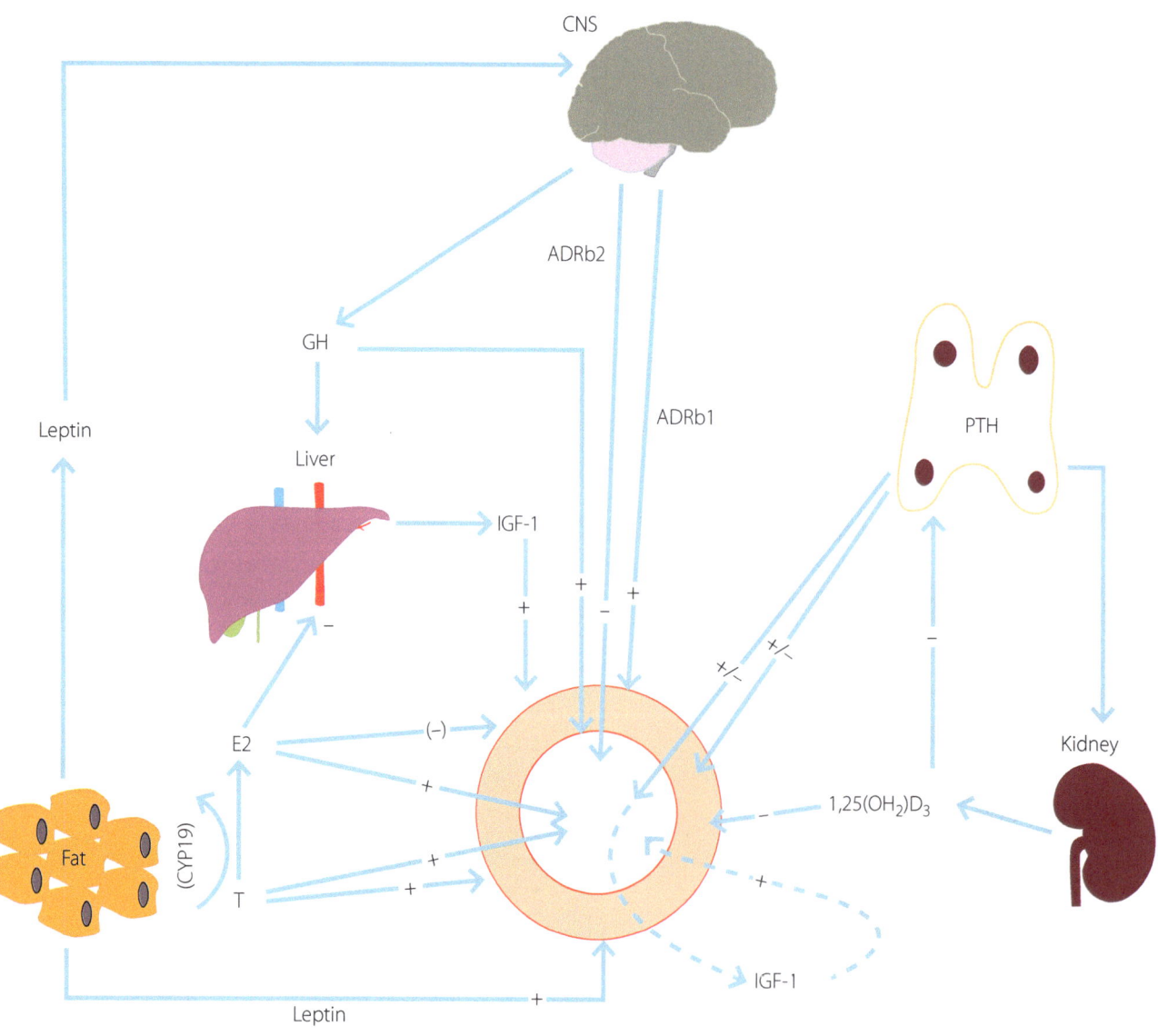

Mineralization of bone tissue

Figure 1.11. The formation of bone is a multistep process, which takes place as part of bone remodeling after bone resorption (see Figure 1.12). The first step in the formation is the synthesis of osteoid, which is laid down at specific sites. After approximately 5–10 days of deposition of this new matrix it begins to mineralize (primary mineral apposition). Once the basic structural matrix is formed a secondary mineralization process begins. The secondary mineralization process is much slower, and is a gradual maturation of the mineral component of the matrix of varying duration. This maturation includes an increase in the number of the hydroxyapatite crystals, and an increase in the size of the crystals to their maximum, plus alterations in their internal order, which reflects their degree of perfection. The degree of mineralization is dependent on the amount of solid protein present. Therefore, various degrees of mineralization can be seen in adult calcified tissues, with enamel having the most mineralization, and lamellar bone the least. DMB, degree of mineralization of bone. Adapted from Boivin G, Meunier PJ. Methodological considerations in measurement of bone mineral content. Osteoporos Int 2003; 14(Suppl 5):S22–S28.

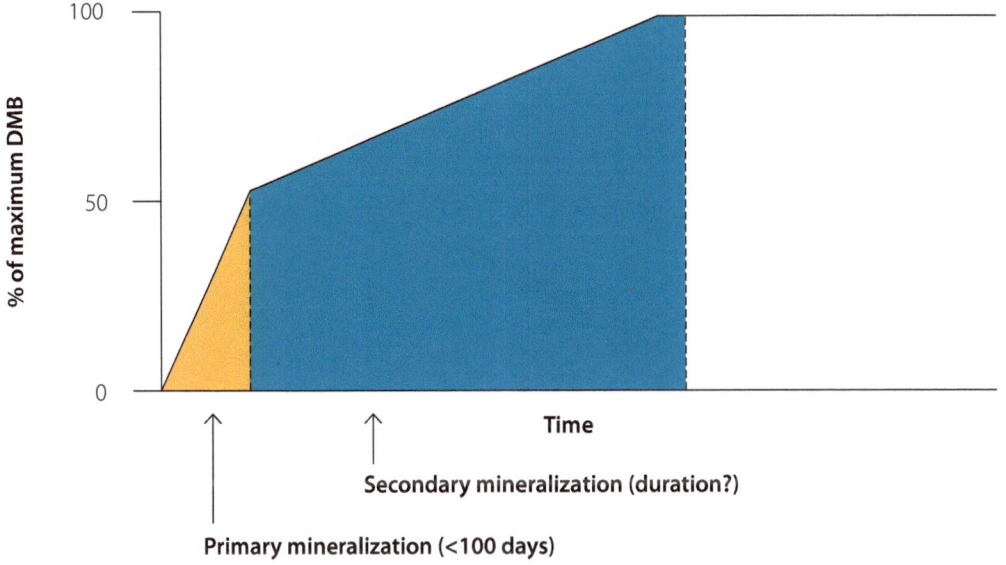

Bone remodeling

Figure 1.12. The mechanical integrity of the skeleton is maintained by the process of bone remodeling, which occurs throughout life. This process of regeneration, degradation, and repair, allows damaged bone to be replaced by new bone. Remodeling can be divided into four phases: resorption, reversal, formation, and quiescence. At any one time, approximately 10% of bone surfaces in the adult skeleton are undergoing active remodeling, whereas the remaining 90% is quiescent. The duration of the remodeling cycle is approximately six months, with the resorption phase taking 10–14 days, and formation approximately 150 days. The process of bone remodeling involves osteoblasts (OBs), the bone-forming cells, and osteoclasts (OCs), the bone-resorbing cells working coordinately in the basic multicellular unit. Osteoclasts are multinucleated cells derived from hematopoietic mononuclear cells (MN). They are responsible for the initial stages of bone remodeling. After OCs have removed a quantum of bone, the reversal phase occurs during which OCs detach from the bone surface (and undergo apoptosis) while OBs differentiate from mesenchymal stem cells found in bone marrow. The OBs line the bone surface, and synthesize osteoid ie, the new bone matrix, in pale blue (S), on the lower panel showing bone histomorphometry of the iliac crest; see also Figure 1.2. Once an osteoblast has synthesized and mineralized osteoid (in purple, M on the lower panel), it may become a lining cell, an osteocyte, or it may undergo apoptosis. Reproduced with permission from Hock JM, Krishnan V, Oniya JE et al. Osteoblast apoptosis and bone turnover. J Bone Miner Res 2001; 16:975–84.

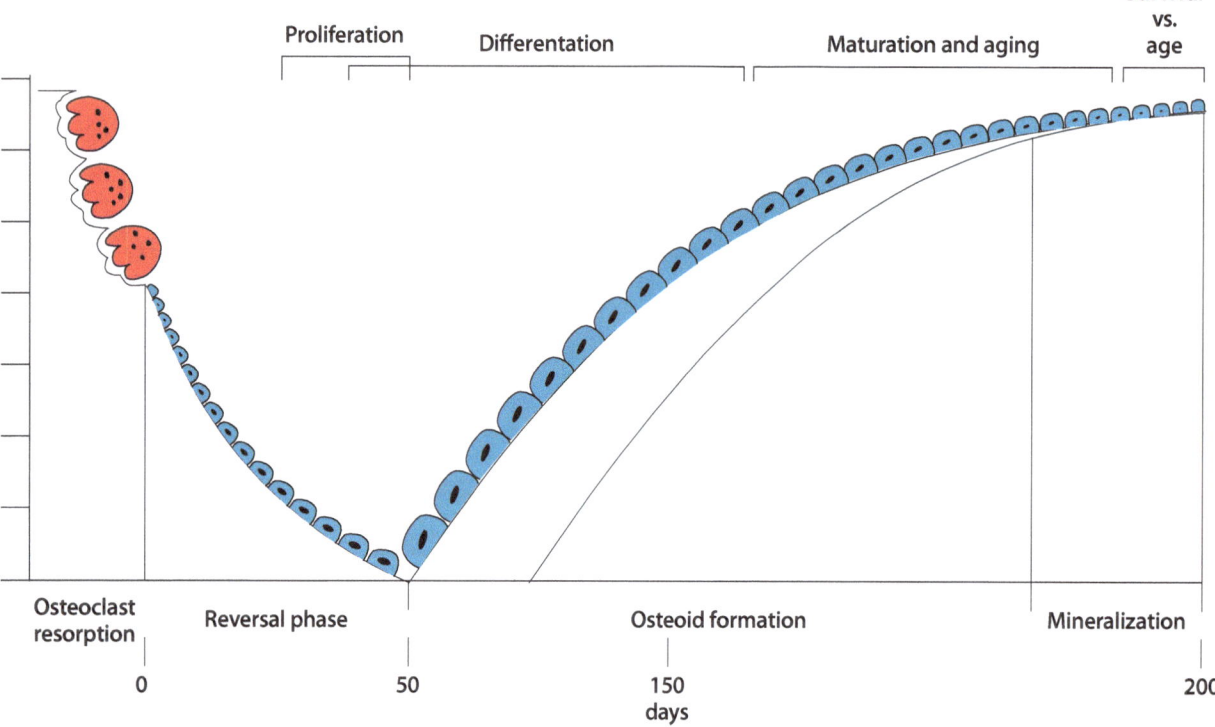

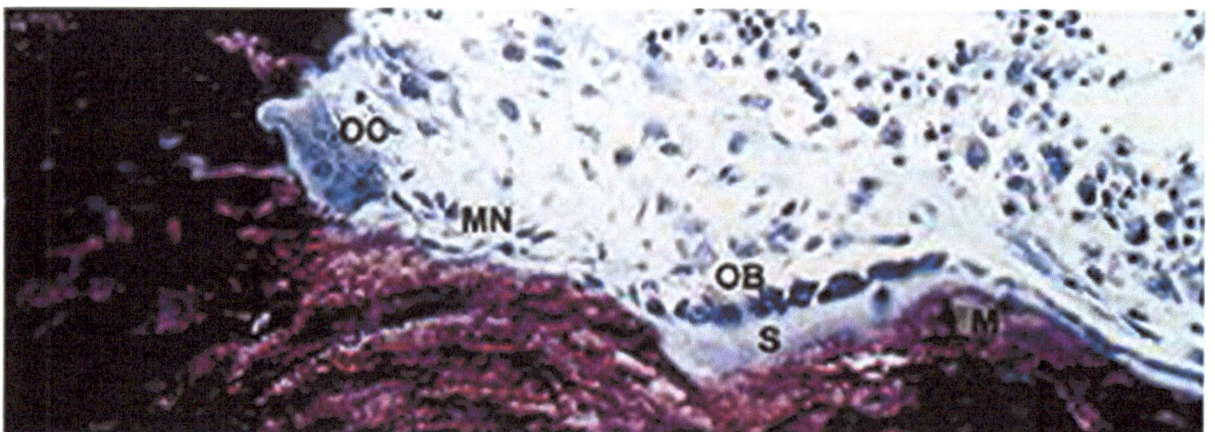

Adolescent changes in bone geometry

Figure 1.13. (a) During adolescence there are changes in bone geometry that accompany gains in bone size and mineral as the medullary cavity expands. There is not only an increase in the size of the vertebrae, but also an increase in the thickness of trabeculae within the bone [Seeman, 2002]. There are also increases in the length and cross-sectional area of long bones. The increases in cortical thickness are largely proportional to the increase in bone diameter, thus the volumetric bone density of long bones changes little throughout childhood and adolescence. During puberty, the hip axial length increases, but the ratio of hip axial length to height does not change [Lee et al. 1997]. These changes are important clinically because bone size and shape influence bone strength, which is independent of bone mineral content [Seeman, 2002]. Adapted from Seeman E. Pathogenesis of bone fragility in women and men. Lancet 2002; 359:1841–50. **(b)** The left hand panel shows the structure of the external cortex (EC) on a transiliac bone specimen: the mineralized bone appears in green, whereas unmineralized tissues, (ie, osteoid surface, OS, periosteum, Ps, and muscle, MM) appear in red. The middle panel illustrates bone formation at the EC in a growing individual, as revealed by the distance between the two fluorescent tetracycline labels. The right hand figure shows the changes in bone formation rate (BFR/BS) during childhood and adolescence, as calculated from tetracycline double labeling. BFR on the external cortex periosteal surface (ECPs) increases several fold during the early stages of puberty, and virtually disappears thereafter, as compared to bone formation on trabecular surfaces (Tb), which is less prominent and more constant throughout growth. Reproduced with permission from Rauch F, Travers R, Glorieux FH. Cellular activity on the seven surfaces of iliac bone: a histomorphometric study in children and adolescents. J Bone Miner Res 2006; 21:513–9.

(a)

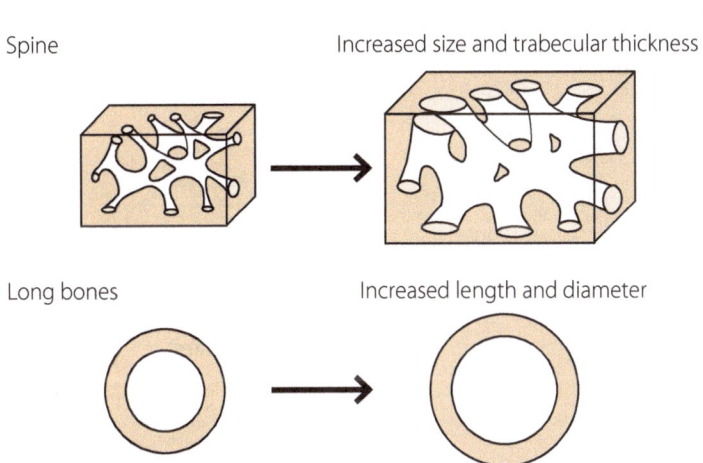

(b)

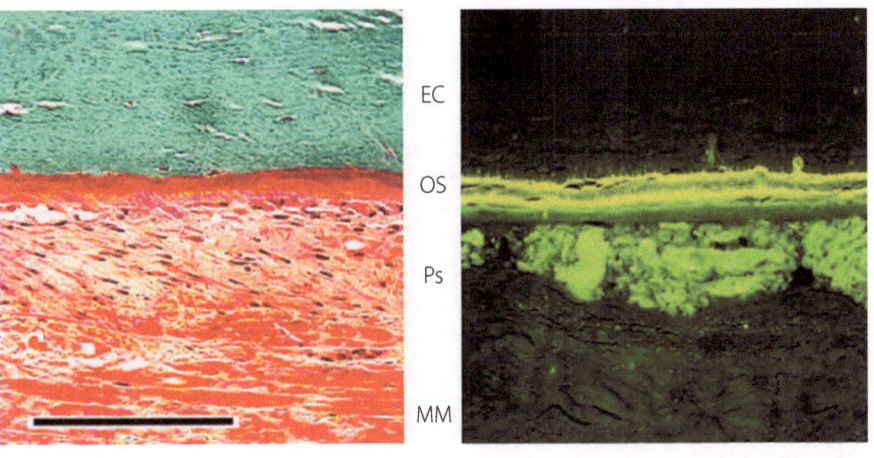
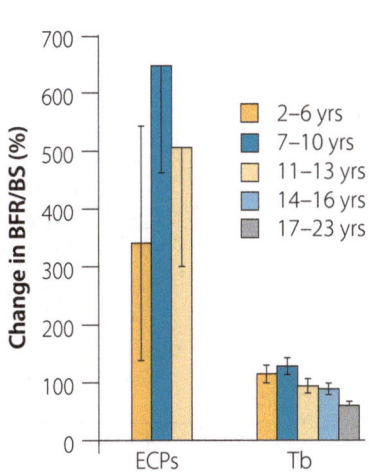

Influence of menarcheal age on bone microstructure

Figure 1.14. Estrogen is essential for normal bone maturation and mineral acquisition. Estrogen can affect chondrocytes, which are responsible for the secretion of extracellular matrix of cartilage. It has been found that patients with rare disorders of estrogen resistance (owing to a mutation in the estrogen receptor), or impaired synthesis (aromatase deficiency) have osteopenia and delayed epiphyseal closure [Bachrach & Smith, 1996]. Skeletal maturation and increases in bone mineral acquisition can be achieved with estrogen therapy [Bilezikian et al. 1998]. It is possible that androgens may also be essential for normal bone mineral accrual and growth, especially for long bones [Wiren & Orwell, 2001]. This figure illustrates that later menarcheal age in healthy females is associated with **(a)** lower areal bone mineral density (aBMD), **(b)** cortical volumetric density and **(c)** thickness at the distal radius, pertaining to a shorter exposure to estradiol (E2) during growth. In turn it may predispose to Colle's fractures after the menopause. Reproduced with permission from Chevalley T, Bonjour JP, Ferrari S et al. Influence of age at menarche on forearm bone microstructure in healthy young women. J Clin Endocrinol Metab 2008; 93:2594–601.

(a)

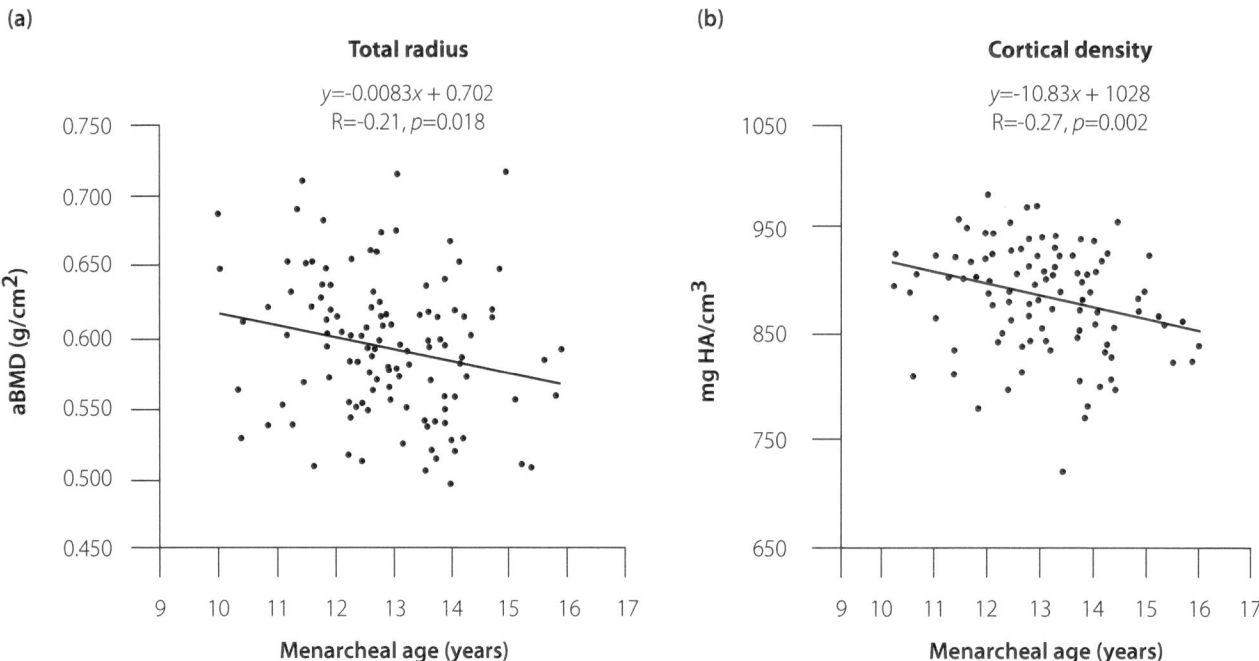

(b)

(c)

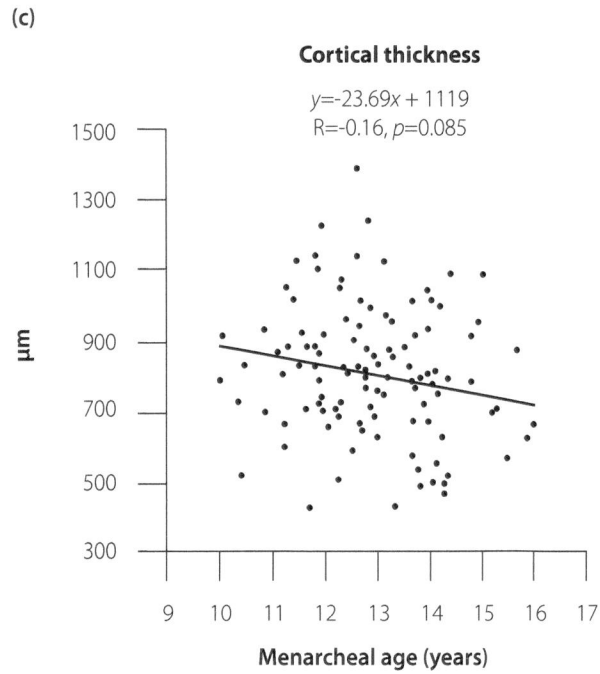

Bone mineral acquisition during puberty

Figure 1.15. From infancy to childhood the total skeletal calcium increases dramatically. Approximately 50% of this increase occurs during adolescence, which makes this period critical in establishing bone health [Bonjour & Rizzoli, 2001; Bailey et al. 1999]. During the second decade peak bone mass is reached, and this serves as the bone bank for the remainder of adult life [Theintz et al. 1992]. The more robust the skeletal mass at its peak, the greater the amount of bone loss (from aging, menopause and other factors) that can be tolerated without clinical signs of osteoporosis. Bone mineral acquisition during adolescence is more closely linked to pubertal development than to chronological age [Bonjour & Rizzoli, 2001; Bailey et al. 1999]. This study measured the changes in lumbar spine (L2–L4), and femoral neck bone mineral density (BMD) using dual-X-ray absorptiometry at one-year intervals in 98 females and 100 males aged 9–19 years. The most rapid increases in the lumbar spine (L2–L4) **(a)**, and femoral neck **(b)**, BMD were between the ages of 11 and 14 years in girls and 14 and 17 years in boys. This result reflects the later onset of puberty in boys, but also a longer period of bone mineral mass acquisition, eventually resulting in a 10–15% greater peak bone mass in the latter. The gains in BMD were greater at the spine and hip than at the forearm or shaft of the femur. The study showed a drastic reduction in bone mass acquisition in healthy girls by the age of 16 years both at the lumbar spine and femoral neck. Girls are known to reach 95% of their adult bone mineral content by the age of 18 years, and have only modest gains during the third decade of life. Adapted from Theintz G, Buchs B, Rizzoli R et al. Longitudinal monitoring of bone mass accumulation in healthy adolescents: evidence for a marked reduction after 16 years of age at the levels of lumbar spine and femoral neck in female subjects. J Clin Endocrinol Metab 1992; 75:1060–5.

(a)

(b)

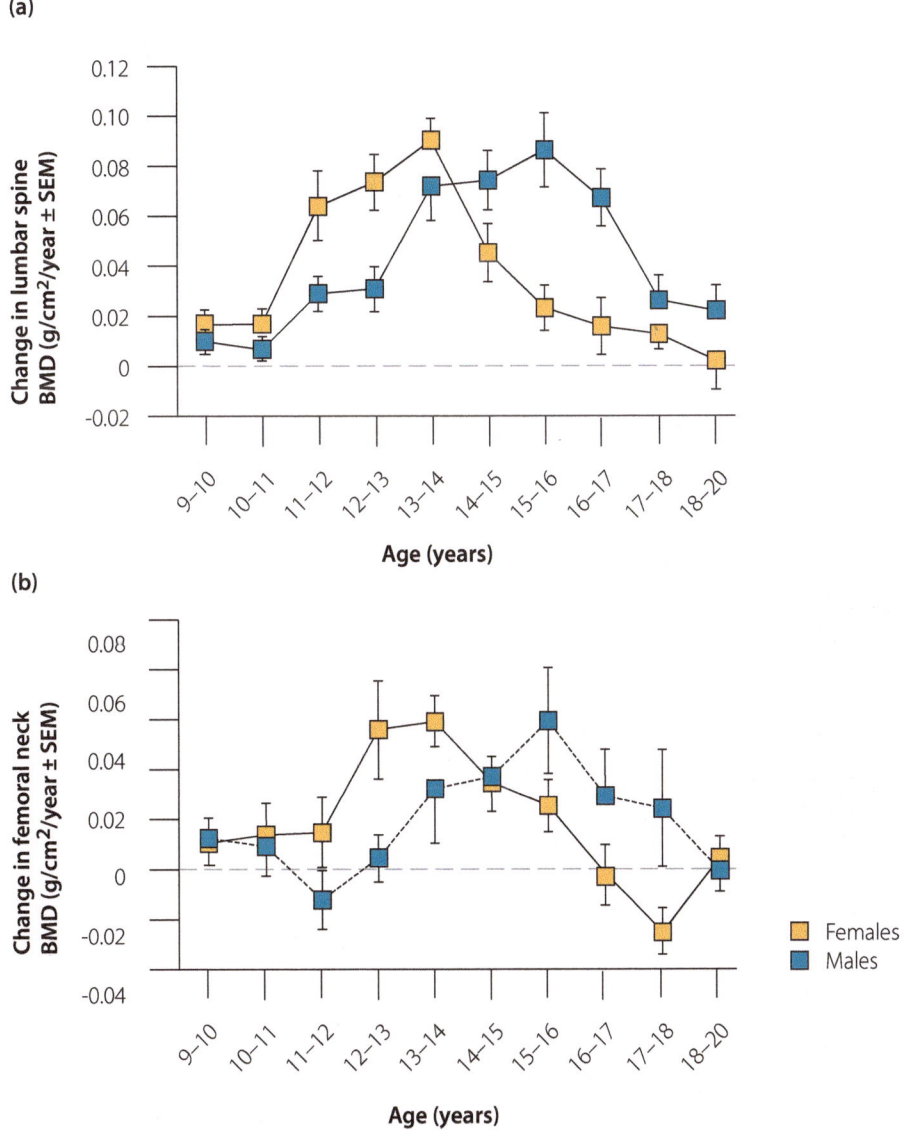

Lifestyle: physical activity is an important stimulus for bone mineral acquisition

Figure 1.16. Physical activity has been shown to be an important stimulus for bone mineral acquisition. It has been found that elite childhood athletes can increase bone size and mineral content during childhood and adolescence [Haaspasalo et al. 1998], and even everyday activities (eg, sports, games, dancing, and physical education classes) can improve bone health. A six-year longitudinal study [Bailey et al. 1999] of 53 girls and 60 boys found that the most active boys and girls gained significantly more bone mineral content (BMC) in the total body (**a**), lumbar spine (**b**), and femoral neck (**c**), during adolescence than did their inactive peers. One year after the peak BMC velocity, there was a 9% and 17% greater total body BMC in boys and girls, respectively, than in their inactive peers. On average, 26% of adult total body BMC was accrued during the two years around peak BMC velocity. *p<0.005; †p<0.001, compared with inactive. Reproduced with permission from Bailey DA, McKay HA, Mirwald RL et al. A six-year longitudinal study of physical activity to bone mineral accrual in growing children: the university of Saskatchewan bone mineral accrual study. J Bone Miner Res 1999; 14:1672–9.

(a) (b)

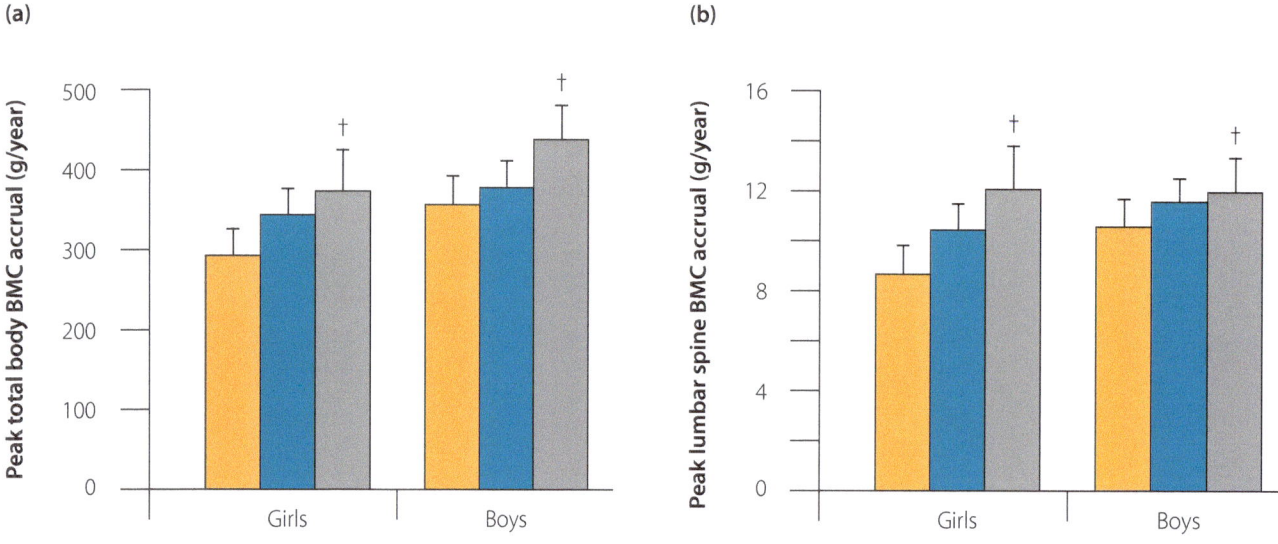

(c)

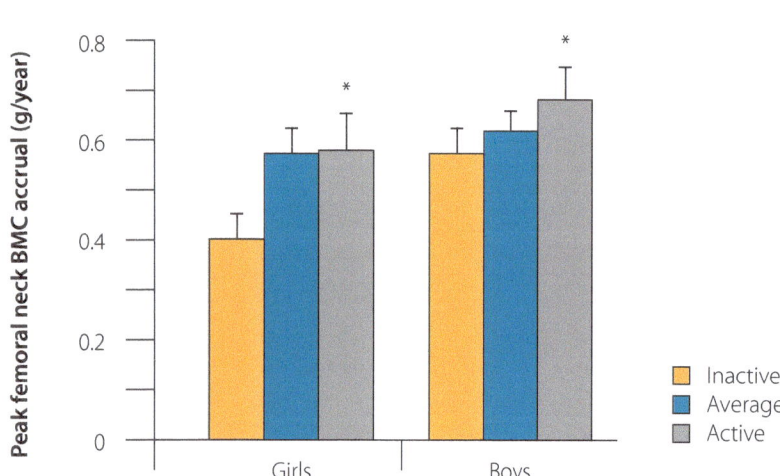

Nutrition: effects of calcium in younger children

Figure 1.17. Evidence from studies in young children has suggested that dietary calcium supplementation is associated with an increase in bone mineral density (BMD). In a double-blind, placebo-controlled study, pre-pubertal, and pubertal, monozygous twins were randomly allocated to receive calcium supplements (calcium citrate malate 1000 mg/day), or placebo, for three years. The children who received the calcium supplements consumed, on average, 1612 mg/day of calcium compared with 908 mg/day in the placebo-treated group. During the study, it was found that the prepubertal twins receiving calcium supplements had higher bone density than those receiving placebo, but there was no benefit of calcium supplements in the pubertal children. It is still not clear whether calcium supplementation has beneficial effects on fracture risk in childhood or later, in adulthood. Adapted from Johnston CC, Miller JZ, Slemenda CW et al. Calcium supplementation and increases in bone mineral density in children. N Engl J Med 1992; 327:82–7.

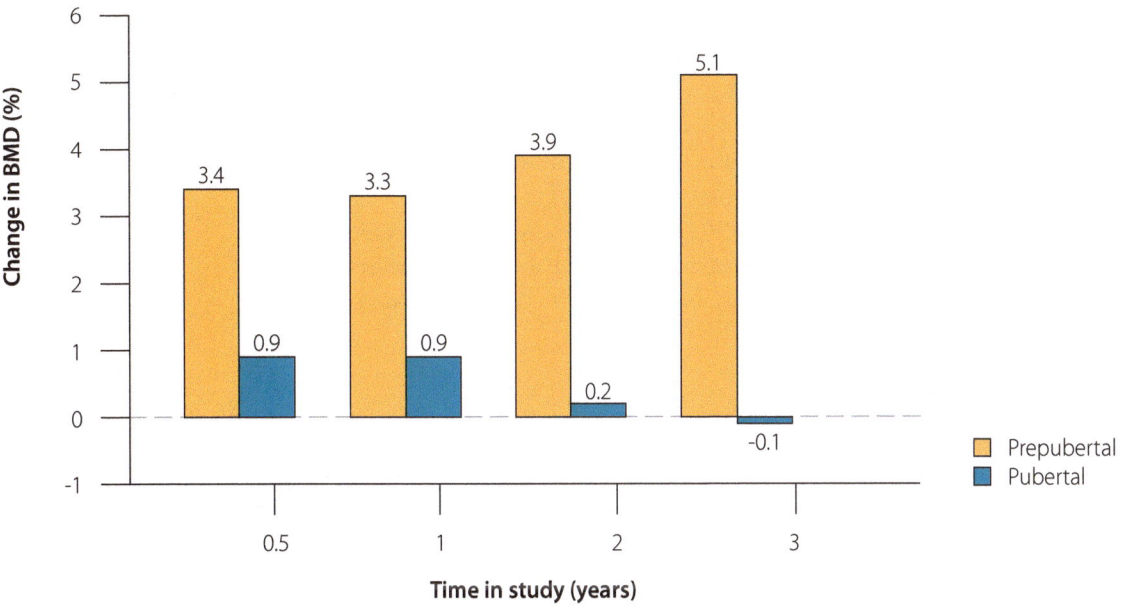

Factors influencing body and bone mass

Figure 1.18. Genetic factors account for 60–80% of the observed variance in adult bone mineral mass. By modulating gene expression levels, gender and hormones, particularly gonadal steroids, have a profound influence on bone mass gain and loss, ultimately resulting in marked differences in the risk of osteoporosis and fragility fractures between men and women. Genetic factors also interact with lifestyle factors (smoking, alcohol, and others) and nutrition (calcium, proteins). In addition, bone accrual and maintenance is stimulated by weight-bearing physical activity, while bone loss is accelerated by immobility. Body mass is highly correlated with bone mass, perhaps because weight reflects bone size, and nutritional status. Body weight may also act as a mechanical load to the skeleton. The lean mass component rather than the fat mass component of total body weight is associated more highly with bone mass. Diseases such as diabetes (mostly type 1), anorexia nervosa and inflammatory bowel disease are associated with lower body mass and/or bone mass through multiple mechanisms.

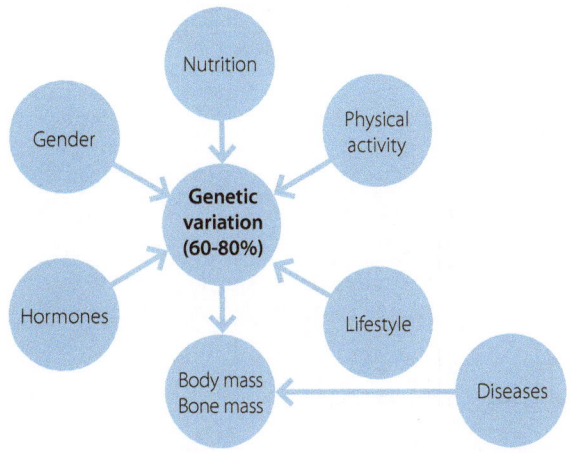

The genetic risk of osteoporosis

Figure 1.19. Single nucleotide polymorphisms (SNPs), variations in the genetic code that do not cause a disease (unlike mutations) but determine the heterogeneity of physical phenotypes among individuals and may predispose to disease, occur at a frequency of 1 every 500–1000 base pairs in the human genome. **(a)** Idiopathic (common) osteoporosis has a strong heritable component, however it is not transmitted according to a Mendelian inheritance pattern (dominant or recessive), as a single gene mutation disorder would be. Rather, susceptibility to osteoporosis is due to a number of SNPs in genes implicated in bone mass acquisition and turnover, each one of these SNPs contributing only a few percent to the genetic risk of osteoporosis in the population, and differing in importance in various populations, this being largely explained by gene-environment interactions. From Ferrari S. Génétique de l'ostéoporose. In: Traité des maladies métaboliques osseuses de l'adulte. Edited by M C de Vernejoul and P Marie. Paris: Flammarion Médecine-Sciences, 2008a. **(b)** This table shows the main genes with polymorphisms within or near the genes that are definitely associated with areal bone mineral density (aBMD) and/or fractures in large population studies. Genome wide association studies (GWAS) that analyse hundreds of thousands of SNPs in each individual represent the strongest hypothesis-free approach to identify genetic variations for common diseases. The genes associated with osteoporosis by GWAS shown here are the first ones to be identified and confirmed by this approach, however these analyses suggest that dozens of other genes are implicated, which still need replication. Consistent results have also been obtained through meta-analyses of multiple association studies focusing on one gene (candidate gene approach), these include: meta-analysis retrospective (MAR), and meta-analysis at participant level (MAP), with (+) or without (-) an association. [1]Association – with BMD, + with fractures. [2]Association + with BMD, - with fractures, except incidental vertebral fractures in women (+). [3]Association + with BMD, - with fractures, men only. Reproduced with permission from Ferrari S. Human genetics of osteoporosis. Best Pract Res Clin Endocrinol Metab 2008b; 22:723–35.

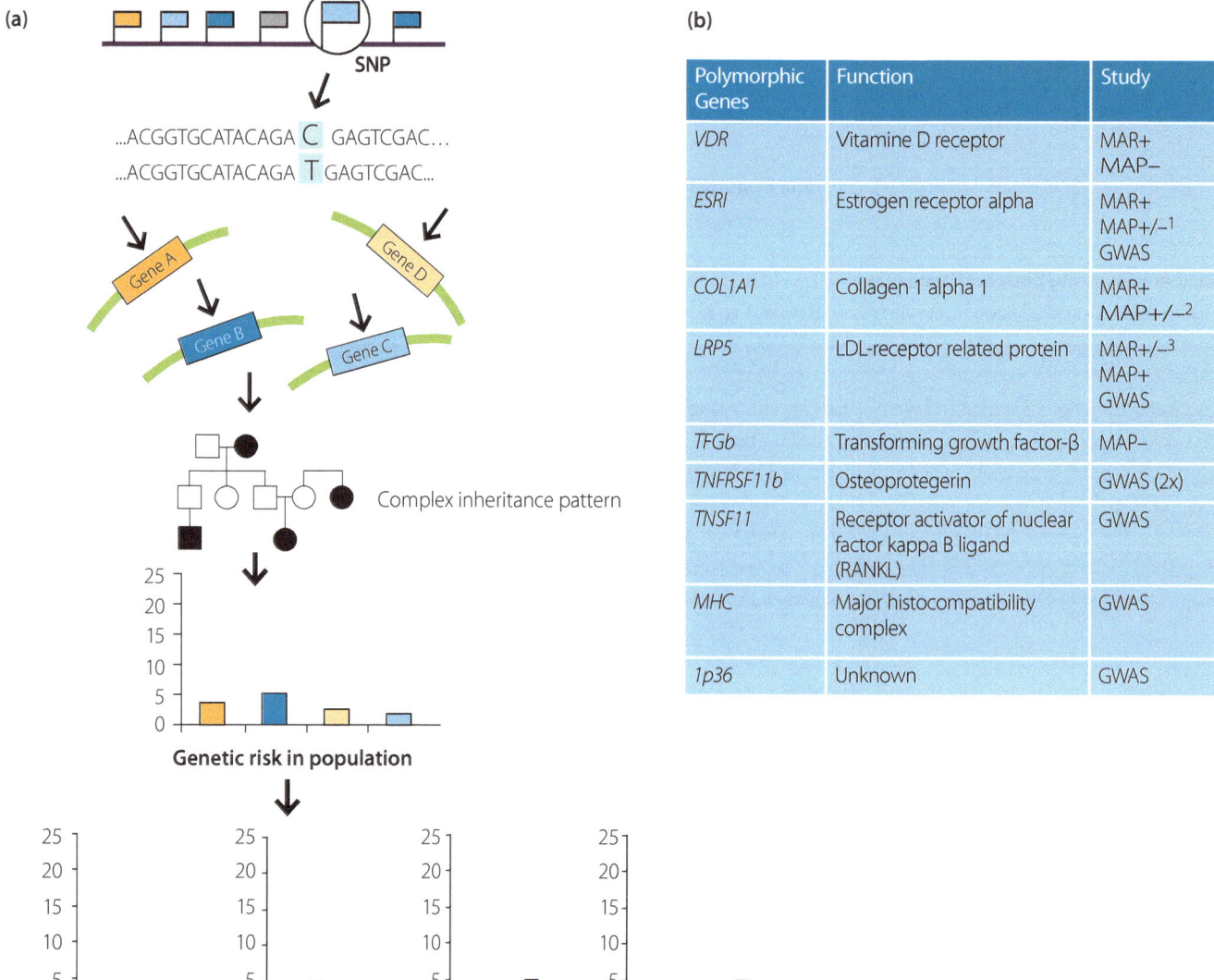

(a)

(b)

Polymorphic Genes	Function	Study
VDR	Vitamine D receptor	MAR+ MAP–
ESRI	Estrogen receptor alpha	MAR+ MAP+/–[1] GWAS
COL1A1	Collagen 1 alpha 1	MAR+ MAP+/–[2]
LRP5	LDL-receptor related protein	MAR+/–[3] MAP+ GWAS
TFGb	Transforming growth factor-β	MAP–
TNFRSF11b	Osteoprotegerin	GWAS (2x)
TNSF11	Receptor activator of nuclear factor kappa B ligand (RANKL)	GWAS
MHC	Major histocompatibility complex	GWAS
1p36	Unknown	GWAS

Bone loss in postmenopausal women

Figure 1.20. Normal trabecular bone is composed of internal beams, or plates, that form a three-dimensional branching lattice, which is orientated along the lines of stress. Trabecular bone has a large surface area, and lies in close proximity to the marrow-derived cells that participate in bone turnover. Bone loss initially starts at the bone surfaces. Therefore, changes in bone mass occur earlier, and to a greater extent, in trabecular bone than in regions of the skeleton that are primarily cortical. **(a)** This figure illustrates the percentage loss of trabecular bone microarchitecture over one year in placebo-treated postmenopausal women, as evaluated by micro-computed tomography of iliac crest bone biopsies. As compared to the 3.3% loss of spine bone mineral density (BMD), there was a disproportionate loss of trabecular number and volume, with a marked increase in the space between trabeculae. The insets illustrate the loss of horizontal struts leading to mechanical failure, as seen in vertebrae or distal radius. Data from Dufresne TE, Chmielewski PA, Manhart MD et al. Risedronate Preserves Bone Architecture in Early Postmenopausal Women In 1 Year as Measured by Three-Dimensional Microcomputed Tomography. Calcif Tissue Int 2003; 73:423–32. Images courtesy of D Dempster. **(b)** This schematic representation further illustrates the cortical bone changes that occur in women: after the menopause, there is cortical thinning by endocortical bone resorption, and cortical porosity from accelerated haversian bone remodeling, without a compensatory periosteal apposition. The estimated changes in cortical thickness (Ct.Th) and volumetric BMD (Ct. vBMD) between age 20 (peak bone mass) and 90 are from cross-sectional measurements obtained by high-resolution computed tomography at the distal radius. Data from Khosla S, Riggs BL, Atkinson EJ et al. Effects of sex and age on bone microstructure at the ultradistal radius: a population-based noninvasive in vivo assessment. J Bone Miner Res 2006; 21:124–31.

(a)

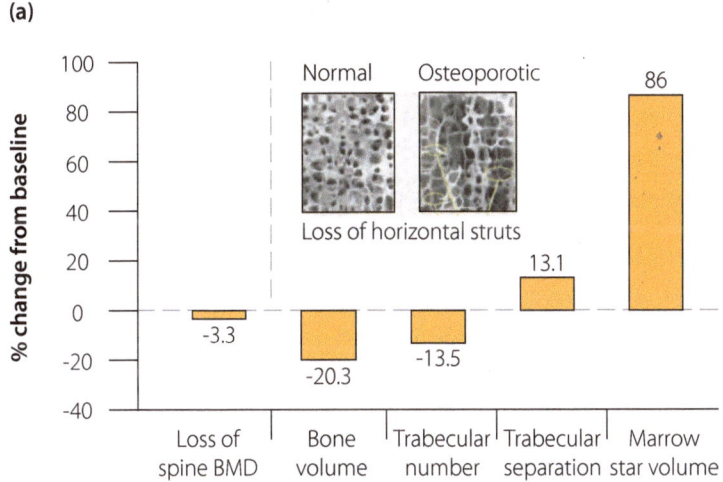

(b)

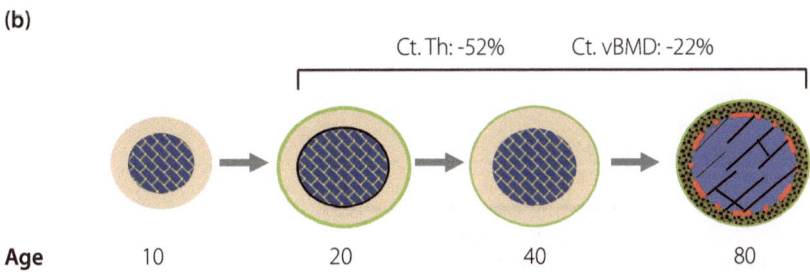

Normal and osteoporotic trabecular structures

Figure 1.21. A comparison of normal (**a**), and osteoporotic (**b**), trabecular structures is shown in these two scanning electron micrographs. In osteoporosis, the trabecular continuity is disrupted by trabecular perforation, and thin rods replace the normal plate-like trabeculae. The qualitative abnormalities in osteoporotic cortical bone are shown in the third microradiograph of a 100 mm thick section from the femoral shaft of a 62- year-old man (**c**). The substantial heterogeneity of the Haversian canal dimensions should be noted. The gray levels indicate patchy differences of mineralization, with white representing the highest level of mineralization. (a) and (b) Courtesy of J Kosek, Stanford University School of Medicine, Stanford, California, USA. (c) Reproduced with permission from Marcus R. The nature of osteoporosis. In: Osteoporosis. Edited by R Marcus, D Feldman, J Kelsey. San Diego: Academic Press, 1996; 647–59.

(a)   (b)   (c)

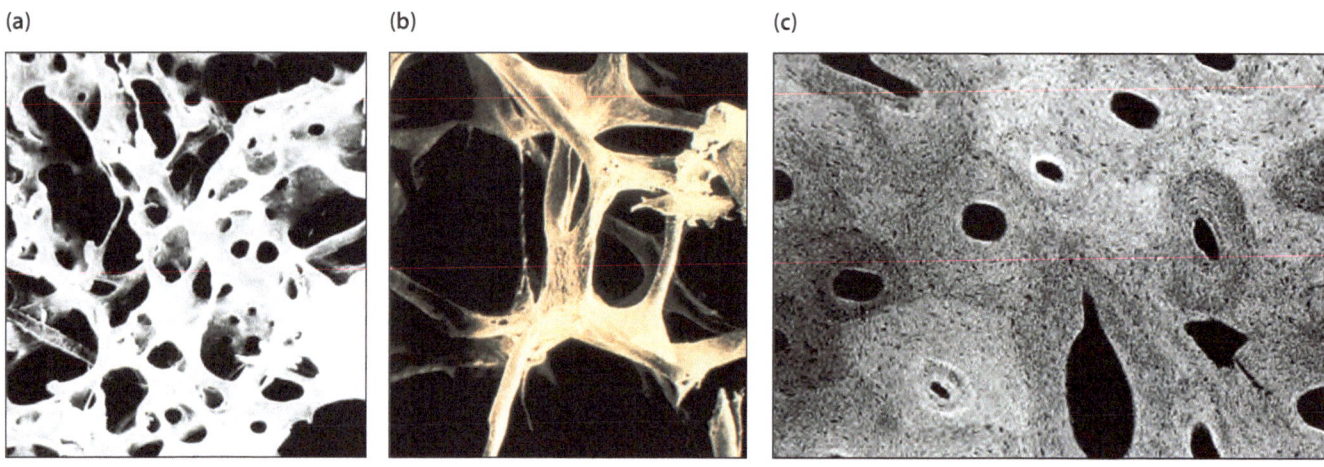

Accelerated bone loss in postmenopausal women

Figure 1.22. Basic mechanisms resulting in accelerated bone loss in postmenopausal women. (**a**) Starting in the perimenopause when menstrual cycles become irregular and culminating at the menopause when ovarian function ceases, levels of estradiol drop abruptly. The activation frequency of remodeling units, that is the speed at which new basic multicellular units (BMUs) are formed on bone surfaces, increases several fold, reaching a maximum in osteoporotic women, as measured here on iliac crest bone biopsies. Data from Recker R, Lappe J, Davies KM et al. Bone remodeling increases substantially in the years after menopause and remains increased in older osteoporosis patients. J Bone Miner Res 2004; 19:1628–33. (**b**) In addition, within each BMU an imbalance occurs between the bone resorbing activity of osteoclasts, which is increased, and the bone forming activity of osteoblasts, which does not quite match bone resorption. The latter may partly be explained by the shorter life span of osteoblasts in the absence of estrogen. Estrogen-deficiency also prompts apoptosis of osteocytes. Reproduced with permission from Ferrari S. Cellular and molecular mechanisms of osteoporosis. In: Innovation in skeletal medicine. Edited by JY Reginster and R Rizzoli. Issy-Les-Moulineaux: Elsevier Masson, 2008c; 19–46.

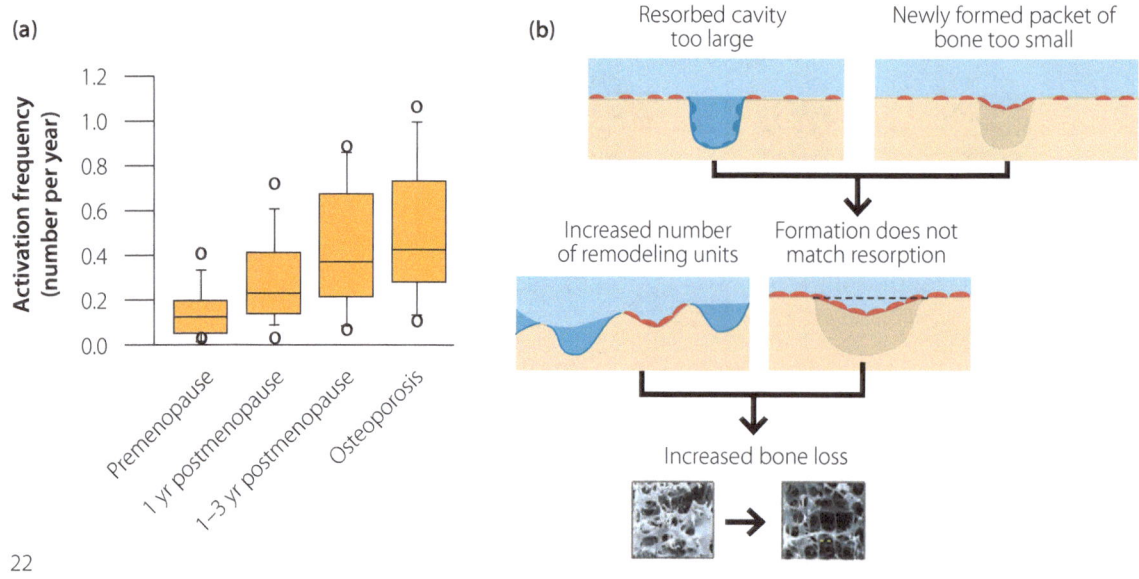

Effect of estrogen and estrogen deficency on bone cells

Figure 1.23. This model illustrates the effect of estrogen (respectively estrogen deficiency) on the intricate crosstalk between immune cells and bone cells by modulating cytokine production in the bone marrow environment. Normally, estrogen supresses (E−) osteoclastogenesis, and induces osteoclast apoptosis (E+) by exerting a direct effect on osteoclasts, bone marrow stromal cells/osteoblasts, monocytes/macrophages and T cells. In particular, estrogen inhibits the production of macrophage colony stimulating factor (M-CSF), receptor activator of nuclear factor kappa B ligand (RANKL) and other osteoclastic cytokines (such as interleukin-6 [IL-6]) and tumor necrosis factor alpha (TNF-α) by osteoblast and/or T lymphocytes, and promote TGF-β inhibitory effects on osteoclasts and T cells. GM-CSF, granulocyte macrophage colony stimulating factor; OPG, osteoprotegerin; PGE$_2$, prostaglandin E$_2$; TGF, transforming growth factor; Reproduced with permission from Clowes JA, Riggs BL, Khosla S et al. The role of the immune system in the pathophysiology of osteoporosis. Immunological Reviews 2005; 208:207–10.

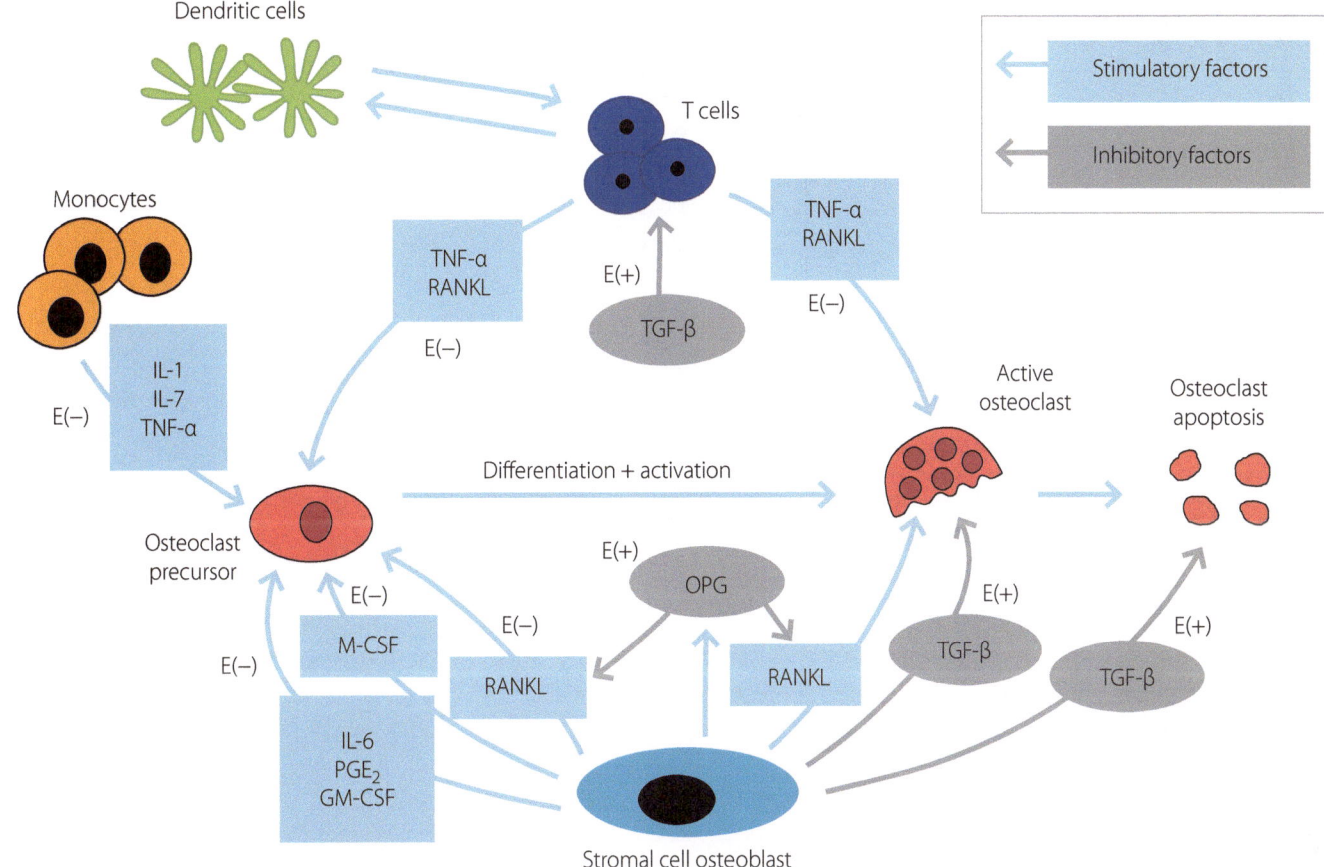

Increased expression of RANKL in postmenopausal women following estrogen deficiency

Figure 1.24. Increased production of the essential osteoclastogenic factor receptor activator of nuclear factor kappa B ligand (RANK)L upon estrogen deficiency is a central mechanism for accelerated bone loss in postmenopausal women. This figure shows that the expression of RANKL at the surface of osteoblast precursors (bone marrow stromal cells), and B and T lymphocytes, as evaluated by the binding of a fluorescent osteoprotegerin (OPG) molecule, is increased threefold in these cells in postmenopausal women compared to premenopausal women. This increase was considerably greater than that associated with hormone replacement. Reproduced with permission from Clowes JA, Riggs BL, Khosla S et al. The role of the immune system in the pathophysiology of osteoporosis. Immunological Reviews 2005; 208:207–10.

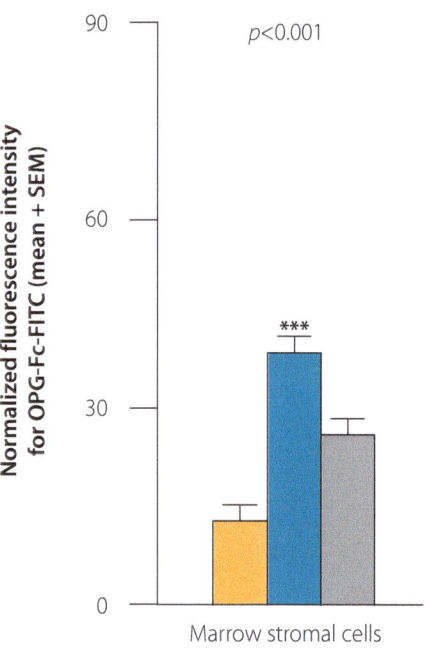
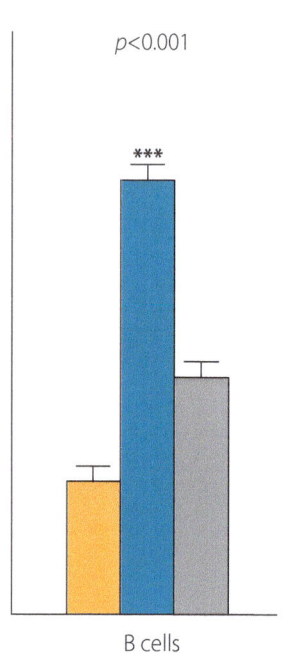

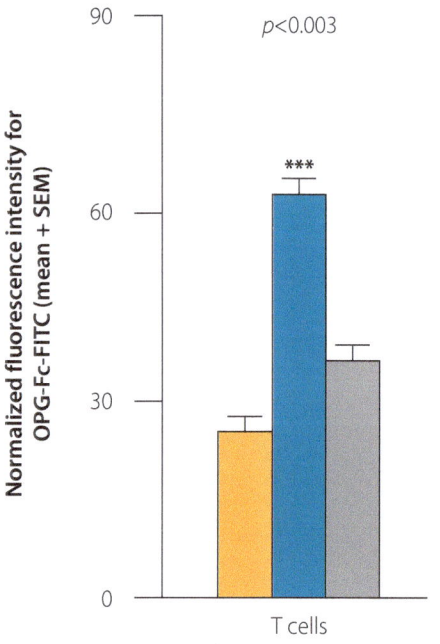
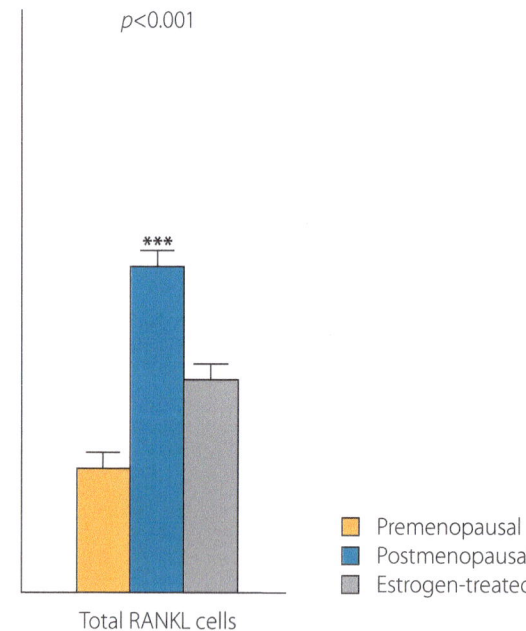

Markers for assessing bone formation and bone resorption

Figure 1.25. In order to measure the rate of bone turnover in osteoporosis a number of specific biochemical markers have been developed in the last 20 years. These markers have been widely used in clinical research, and in clinical trials, to evaluate efficacy and mechanisms of action of new treatments. These new markers listed above are more sensitive than conventional markers of bone turnover. The markers can be divided into two categories: those for measuring bone formation, and those for bone resorption, although some markers may reflect both. It should be noted that these markers are not disease specific, and will measure alterations in skeletal metabolism regardless of the underlying cause. The markers of bone formation detect direct, or indirect, products of active osteoblasts, which are expressed at different phases of development, and reflect osteoblast function and bone formation. These markers are measured in the serum, or plasma. The markers for bone resorption are generally degradation products of collagen, but markers for noncollagenous proteins are also being investigated. Adapted from Delmas PD, Eastell R, Garnero P et al. The use of biochemical markers of bone turnover in osteoporosis. Osteoporos Int 2000; 11(Suppl 6):S2–S17.

Bone formation markers	Comments about assay
Osteocalcin Osteocalcin (or bone-Gla-protein [BGP]) Undercarboxylated osteocalcin Total osteocalcin Intact osteocalcin N-mid fragment of osteocalcin	Intact + N-mid fragment
Alkaline phosphatase Total alkaline phosphatase Bone specific alkaline phosphatase	Bone + liver + other sources
Type 1 collagen propeptides Procollagen type 1 N propeptide Monomer of procollagen type 1 N propeptide Intact procollagen type 1 N propeptide Total procollagen type 1 N propeptide Procollagen type 1 C propeptide	Also called extension peptides of type 1 collagen Refers to trimer Monomer + trimer
Bone resorption markers	
Hydroxyproline Hydroxylysine Galactosyl hydroxylysine Glucosyl galactosyl hydroxylysine Pyridinoline Deoxypyridinoline	} Total (ie, free + peptide-bound) urinary excretion unless otherwise specified Urinary excretion of free moieties unless otherwise specified Can be qualified by total, free moieties or peptide-bound and in serum and urine
Type 1 collagen telopeptides N-terminal cross-linking telopeptide of type 1 collagen C-terminal cross-linking telopeptide of type 1 collagen C-terminal cross-linking telopeptide of type 1 collagen generated by MMPs	Beta isomerized unless otherwise specified
Bone sialoprotein Acid phosphatase Tartrate-resistant acid phosphatase	Includes two isoforms: type 5a (platelets and other sources) and type 5b (osteoclasts)

Effect of aging and the menopause on bone resorption and formation

Figure 1.26. Changes in the metabolism of bone with aging are responsible for bone loss and osteoporosis. This study investigated the levels of bone formation and bone resorption markers in perimenopausal women (peri MP), and in early (early pMP; within 10 years of the menopause) and late (late pMP; 10 or more years after menopause) postmenopausal women. **(a)** Bone formation was studied using markers of serum osteocalcin, serum bone-specific alkaline phosphatase, and serum C-propeptide of type I collagen (PICP). **(b)** Bone resorption was studied by measuring the urinary excretion of two pyridinoline cross-linked peptides (type 1 cross-linked N-telopeptides [NTX], and type 1 C-telopeptide breakdown products [CTX]). The mean levels for each marker in each group are expressed as a percentage and standard error of the mean over the premenopausal women (pre MP). The T-score is the mean of individual values of early postmenopausal women expressed as the number of standard deviations from the premenopausal mean. The study showed that there were marked increases in both markers of bone formation and bone resorption in the first years following menopause, and that these high levels were maintained in elderly women for up to 40 years after menopause. The high bone turnover, therefore, seems to be an important determinant of bone loss with increasing postmenopausal age. *$p<0.01$, †$p<0.001$ versus pre MP. Reproduced with permission from Garnero P, Sornay-Rendu E, Chapuy M et al. Increased bone turnover in late postmenopausal women is a major determinant of osteoporosis. J Bone Miner Res 1996; 11:337–49.

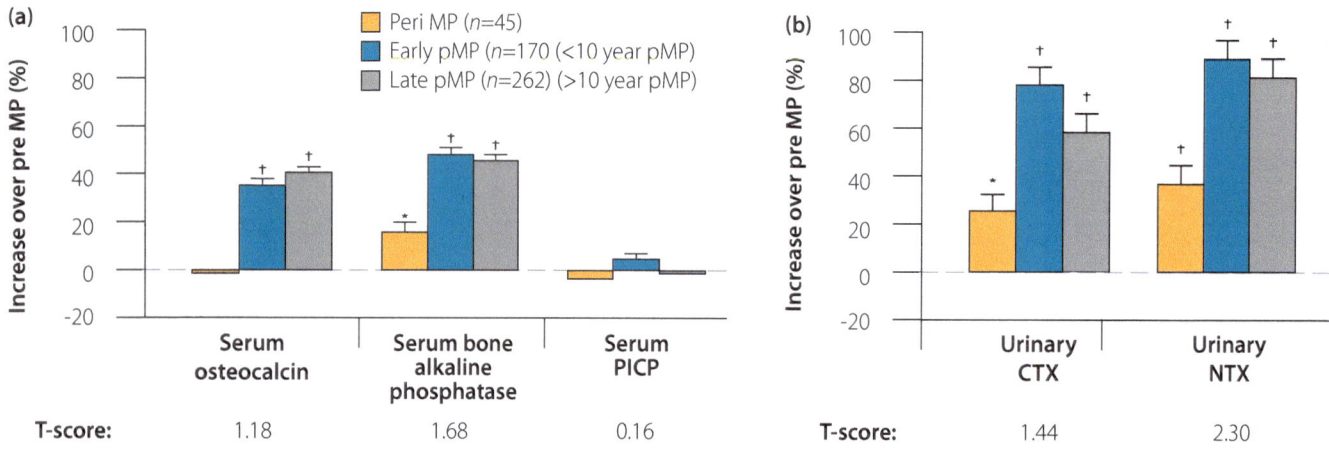

Importance of early bone loss and its association with estrogen deficiency

Figure 1.27. It is well known that there is a decline in bone mass with increasing number of years after the menopause. The importance of early bone loss and its association with estrogen deficiency was investigated in this study by examining the relationship between the number of years since menopause and the rates of bone loss. The longitudinal data for spontaneous loss of lumbar and femoral neck bone mineral density (BMD) in women receiving placebo (n=71; mean age 56.3±4.4 years) were combined from two randomized, controlled trials. The highest rates of bone loss were found in women closest to the menopause. There was a significant relationship between the number of years since menopause and BMD loss at the spine (r=0.34; $p<0.01$) and femoral neck (r=0.25; $p<0.001$). Adapted with permission from Bjarnason NH, Alexandersen P, Christiansen C. Number of years since menopause: spontaneous bone loss is dependent but response to hormone replacement therapy is independent. Bone 2002; 30:637–42.

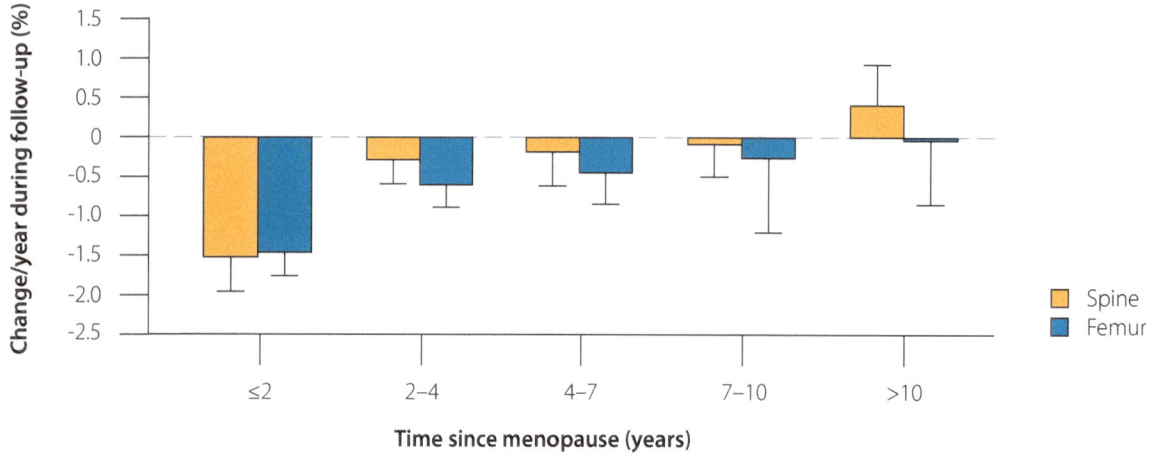

Estrogen replacement after menopause

Figure 1.28. One of the first studies to show that estrogen can prevent, or slow, bone loss, and may modestly increase bone mineral density, whenever it is initiated, was the landmark trial by Lindsay et al. (1976). This was a prospective, double-blind trial that investigated the effects of long-term treatment with estrogen replacement therapy (24.8 mg mestranol, a formulation that is no longer widely used in postmenopausal women), or placebo in 120 women. The women were divided into three groups, those who began therapy two months, three years, or six years after ovariectomy for benign pelvic disease in their late 40s. In a post-hoc analysis, the long-term (>10 years) use of estrogen replacement therapy was found to significantly reduce the rate of loss of metacarpal bone mineral content. The study also showed that the earlier the treatment was begun, the more beneficial its effect on bone loss, as bone that was already lost could not be replaced to any significant extent. Reproduced with permission from Lindsay R, Aitken JM, Anderson JB et al. Long-term prevention of postmenopausal osteoporosis by oestrogen: evidence for an increased bone mass after delayed onset of oestrogen treatment. Lancet 1976; 1:1038–41.

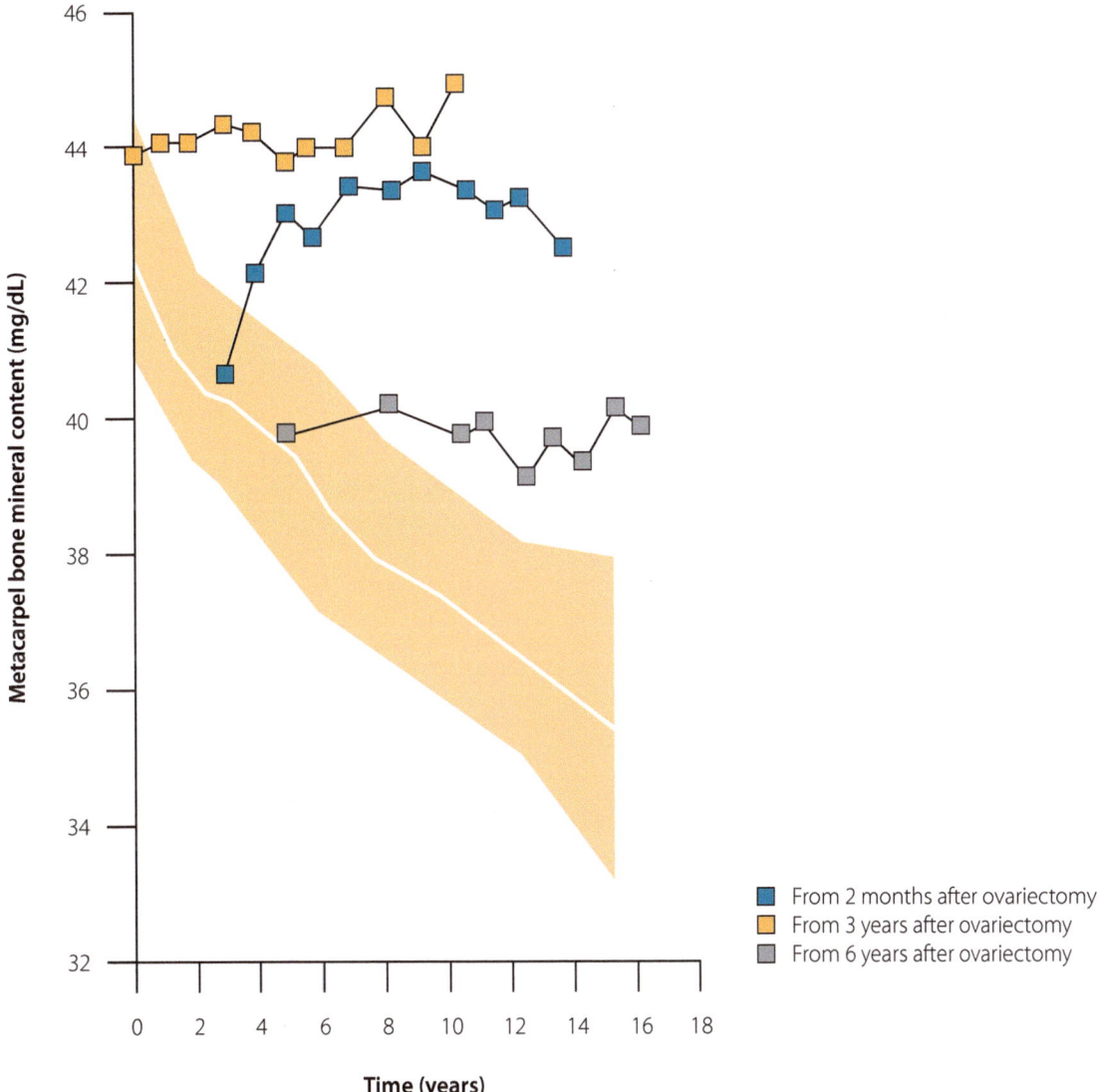

■ From 2 months after ovariectomy
■ From 3 years after ovariectomy
■ From 6 years after ovariectomy

Effects of glucocorticoids on bone remodeling

Figure 1.29. Glucocorticoid excess, either endogenously (such as in Cushing's disease) or exogeneously (use of prednisone in inflammatory conditions), represents a major risk factor for osteoporosis. Glucocorticoids affect bone metabolism both systemically, by directly inhibiting intestinal calcium absorption (thereby competing with vitamin D) and suppressing the production of growth hormone GH/IGF-1 and gonadal steroids, and locally by directly inhibiting the function of osteoblasts and osteocytes while promoting osteoclastic bone resorption, the latter through an increase of RANKL/OPG ratio in the bone marrow environment. CSF, colony stimulating factor; OPG, osteoprotegerin; RANKL, receptor activator of nuclear factor kappa B ligand. Reproduced with permission from Canalis E, Mazziotti G, Giustina A et al. Glucocorticoid-induced osteoporosis: pathophysiology and therapy. Osteoporosis Int 2007; 18:1319–28.

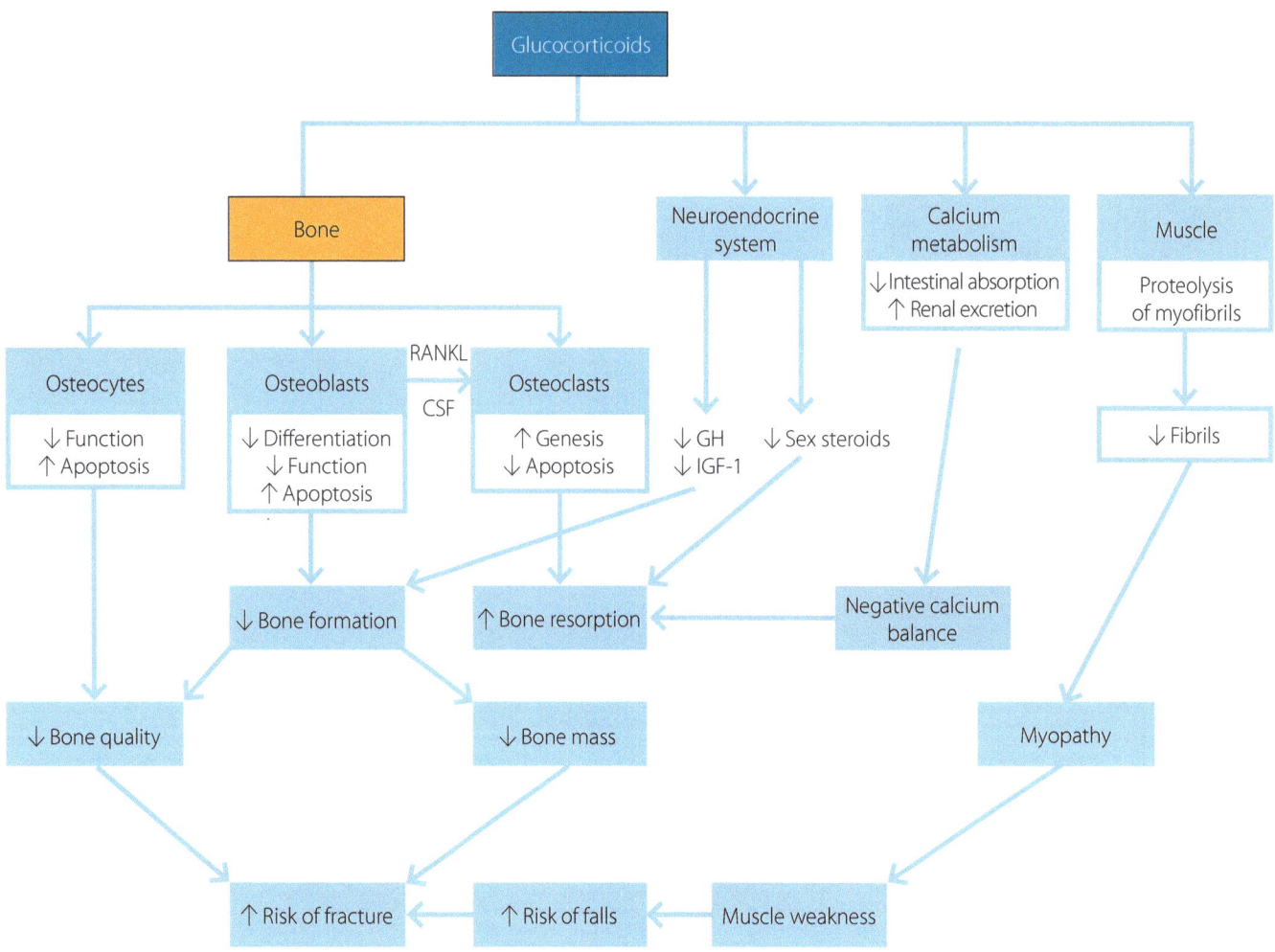

Role of dietary factors in early postmenopausal bone loss

Figure 1.30. One of the factors linked with bone loss occurring close to the menopause is dietary calcium. The principal factor is, however, estrogen deficiency, which increases extracellular calcium concentrations, and consequently suppresses renal calcium reabsorption and gut calcium absorption via effects on parathyroid hormone (PTH) and calcitriol (the major active metabolite of vitamin D). Bone loss itself is, therefore, the main cause of the low gut calcium absorption and high renal calcium excretion. In certain circumstances, a low dietary calcium, or high urine sodium, can exacerbate these losses and induce further bone loss. Data from Riggs BL, Khosla S, Melton JL 3rd. Sex steroids and the construction and conservation of the adult skeleton. Endocr Rev 2002 23:279–302.

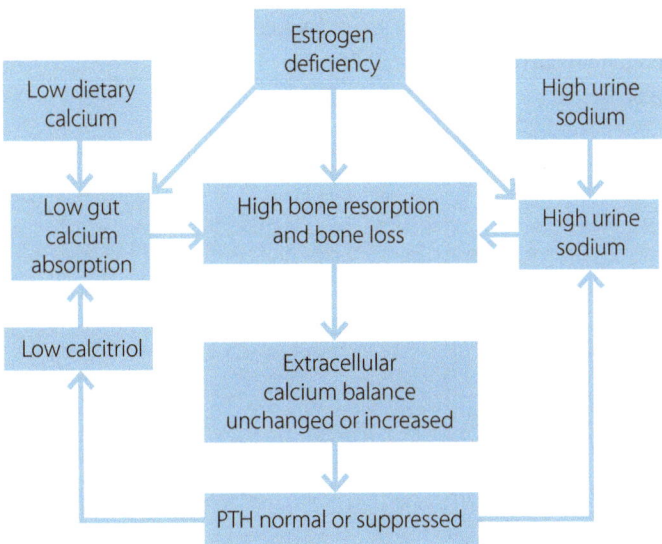

Calcium and estrogen replacement in postmenopausal women

Figure 1.31. The effects of three approaches (exercise, exercise plus calcium supplementation, and exercise plus estrogen replacement therapy) were studied in 120 postmenopausal women who had low forearm bone mineral density. The results showed that in women less than 10 years after the menopause, calcium supplementation prevented forearm bone loss, but estrogen replacement increased bone mass slightly, and was more effective than calcium alone. This study, therefore, demonstrates that calcium is effective, but is less effective than estrogen. Adapted from Prince RL, Smith M, Dick IM et al. Prevention of postmenopausal osteoporosis: a comparative study of exercise, calcium supplementation, and hormone replacement therapy. N Engl J Med 1991; 325:1189–95.

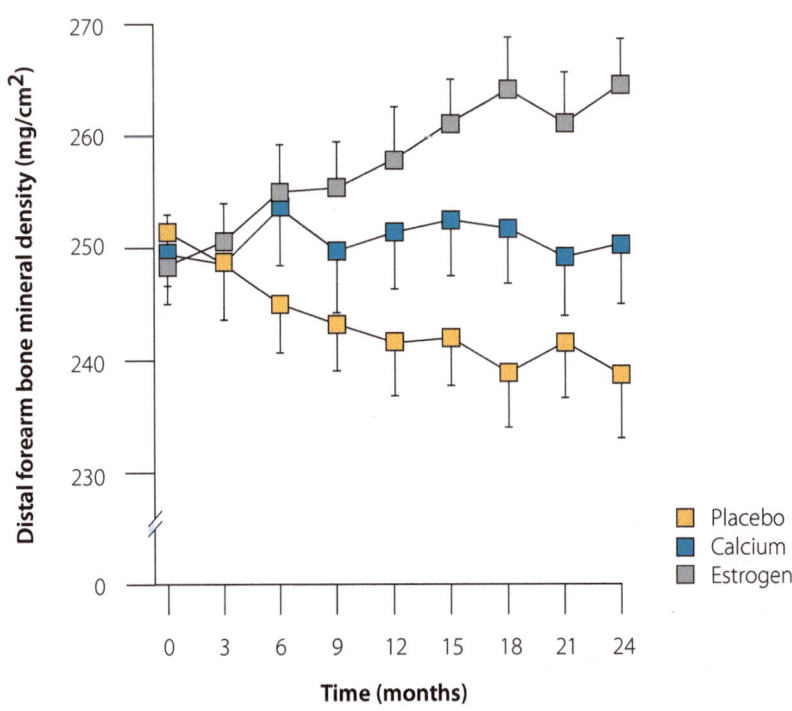

Effects of protein deficiency in elderly patients

Figure 1.32. Protein deficiency, for example, through malnutrition, can contribute to the occurrence of osteoporotic fractures. A protein intake below the recommended daily allowance can result in failure to achieve peak bone mass, and in lack of preservation of bone mass during aging. There is an increased risk of osteoporotic fractures, owing not only to decreased bone mass, but also to an increased propensity to fall because of altered muscle function (eg, lack of strength) and impairment of movement coordination, and of the protective mechanisms against falling, such as reaction times. In addition, the soft tissue is not thick enough to cushion the bones effectively, which increases the mechanical load placed on the osteoporotic bones. The effects of protein deficiency may be mediated through the somatomedin system (insulin-like growth factor-1 [IGF-1]). The figure shows the possible effects of IGF-1 on muscle, bone, fracture risk, and incidence of postfracture medical complications. Adapted from Rizzoli R, Ammann P, Chevalley T et al. Protein intake and bone disorders in the elderly. Joint Bone Spine 2001; 68:383–92.

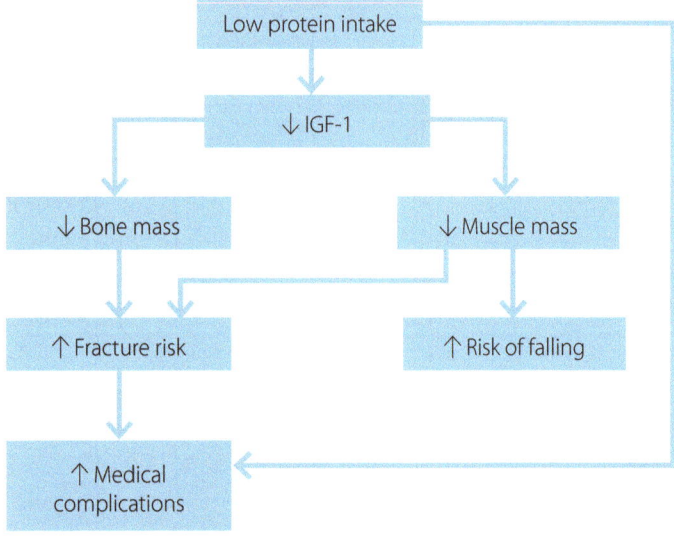

Role of vitamin D in postmenopausal osteoporosis

Figure 1.33. By increasing intestinal absorption of calcium, vitamin D plays a major role on serum calcium homeostasis and bone mineralization. Low levels of vitamin D resulting from poor sun exposure and the age-related decline of synthesis in the skin is extremely frequent in postmenopausal women with osteoporosis, resulting in secondary hyperparathyroidism which may be aggravated by insufficient dietary intake of calcium (ie, below 800 mg/day). Vitamin D insufficiency also causes muscle weakness, and impairs gait and balance, resulting in falls and fractures. In turn, vitamin D supplements of 800 IU/day have been shown to reduce falls and hip fractures by 15–25%, respectively, most efficiently in institutionalized elderly women. PTH, parathyroid hormone.

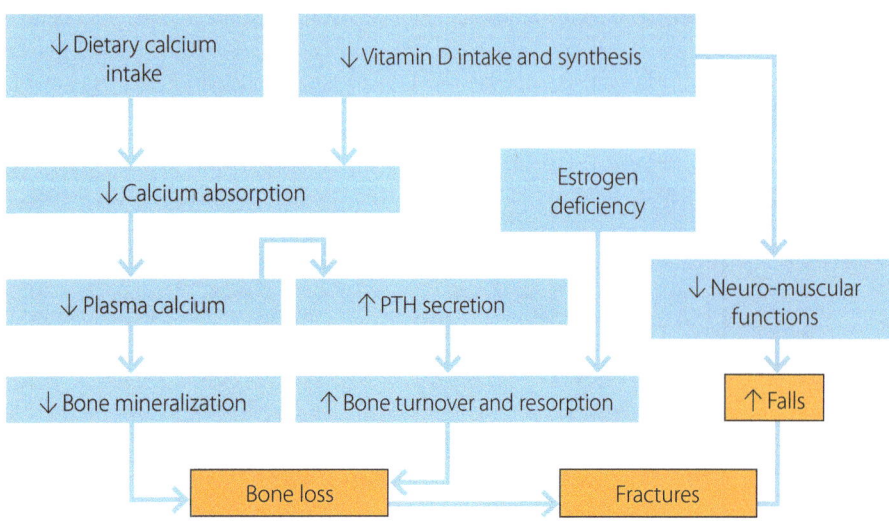

References

Bachrach BE, Smith EP. The role of sex steroids in bone growth and development: evolving new concepts. Endocrinologist 1996; 6:362–8.

Bailey DA, McKay HA, Mirwald RL et al. A six-year longitudinal study of the relationship of physical activity to bone mineral accrual in growing children: the University of Saskatchewan bone mineral accrual study. J Bone Miner Res Oct 1999; 14:1672–9.

Baron R, Rawadi G. Targeting the Wnt/beta-catenin pathway to regulate bone formation in the adult skeleton. Endocrinology 2007; 148:2635–43.

Bilezikian JP, Morishima A, Bell J et al. Increased bone mass a result of estrogen therapy in a man with aromatase deficiency. N Engl J Med 1998; 339:599–603.

Bischoff–Ferrari HA, Willett WC et al. Fracture prevention with vitamin D supplementation: a meta-analysis of randomized controlled trials. JAMA 2005; 293:2257–64.

Bjarnarson NH, Alexandersen P, Christiansen C. Number of years since menopause: spontaneous bone loss is dependent but response to hormone replacement therapy is independent. Bone 2002; 30: 637–42.-

Boivin G, Meunier PJ. Methodological considerations in measurement of bone mineral content. Osteoporos Int 2003; 14(Suppl 5):S22–8.

Bonewald LF. Osteocytes as dynamic multifunctional cells. Ann N Y Acad Sci 2007; 1116:281–90.

Bonjour JP, Rizzoli R. Bone acquisition in adolescence. In: Osteoporosis, volume 1, 2nd edition. Edited by R Marcus, J Kelsey, D Feldman. San Diego: Academic Press, 2001; 621–38.

Bonnet N, Pierroz DD, Ferrari SL. Adrenergic control of bone remodeling and its implications for the treatment of osteoporosis. J Musculoskelet Neuronal Interact 2008; 8:94–104.

Boyle WJ, Simonet WS, Lacey DL. Osteoclast differentiation and activation. Nature 2003; 423:337–342.

Canalis E, Mazziotti G, Giustina A et al. Glucocorticoid-induced osteoporosis: pathophysiology and therapy. Osteoporos Int 2007; 18:1319–28.

Chapuy MC, Arlot ME, Duboeuf F et al. Vitamin D3 and calcium to prevent hip fractures in the elderly women. N Engl J Med 1992; 327:1637–42.

Chevalley T, Bonjour JP, Ferrari S et al. Influence of age at menarche on forearm bone microstructure in healthy young women. J Clin Endocrinol Metab 2008; 93:2594–601.

Christiansen C, Christensen MS, McNair PL et al. Prevention of early menopausal bone loss: conducted 2-year study. Eur J Clin Invest 1980; 10:273–9.

Clowes JA, Riggs BL, Khosla S et al. The role of the immune system in the pathophysiology of osteoporosis. Immunological Reviews 2005; 208: 207–27.

Cohen MM, Jr. The new bone biology: pathologic, molecular, and clinical correlates. Am J Med Genet A 2006; 140:2646–706.

Compston JE. Sex steroids and bone. Physiol Rev 2001; 81:419–447.

Consensus Development Conference. Diagnosis, prophylaxis and treatment of osteoporosis. Am J Med 1993; 94:646–50.

Delmas PD, Eastell R, Garnero P et al. The use of biochemical markers of bone turnover in osteoporosis. Osteoporos Int 2000; 11(Suppl 6):S2–17.

Dufresne TE, Chmielewski PA, Manhart MD et al. Risedronate Preserves Bone Architecture in Early Postmenopausal Women In 1 Year as Measured by Three-Dimensional Microcomputed Tomography. Calcif Tissue Int 2003; 73:423–32.

Eghbali–Fatourechi G, Khosla S, Sanyal A et al. Role of RANK ligand in mediating increased bone resorption in early postmenopausal women. J Clin Invest 2003; 111:1221–30.

Ferrari S. Génétique de l'ostéoporose. In: Traité des maladies métaboliques osseuses de l'adulte. Edited by M C de Vernejoul and P Marie. Paris: Flammarion Médecine-Sciences, 2008a.

Ferrari S. Human genetics of osteoporosis. Best Pract Res Clin Endocrinol Metab 2008b; 22:723–35.

Ferrari S. Cellular and molecular mechanisms of osteoporosis. In: Innovation in skeletal medicine. Edited by JY Reginster and R Rizzoli. Issy-Les-Moulineaux: Elsevier Masson, 2008c; 19–46.

Ferrari SL, Deutsch S, Antonarakis SE. Pathogenic mutations and polymorphisms in the lipoprotein receptor-related protein 5 reveal a new biological pathway for the control of bone mass. Curr Opin Lipidol 2005; 16:207–14.

Garnero P, Sornay-Rendu E, Chapuy M et al. Increased bone turnover in late postmenopausal women is a major determinant of osteoporosis. J Bone Miner Res 1996; 11:337–49.

Goltzman D. Studies on the mechanisms of the skeletal anabolic action of endogenous and exogenous parathyroid hormone. Arch Biochem Biophys 2008; 473:218–24.

Haaspasalo H, Kannus P, Sievannen H et al. Effect of long-term unilateral activity on bone mineral density of female junior tennis players. J Bone Miner Res 1998; 13:310–9.

Hamrick MW, Ferrari SL. Leptin and the sympathetic connection of fat to bone. Osteoporos Int 2008; 19:905–12.

Heino TJ, Hentunen TA. Differentiation of osteoblasts and osteocytes from mesenchymal stem cells. Curr Stem Cell Res Ther 2008; 3:131–45.

Hock JM, .Krishnan V, Oniya JE et al. Osteoblast apoptosis and bone turnover. J Bone Miner Res 2001; 16:975–84.

Hofbauer LC, Gori F, Riggs BL et al. Stimulation of osteoprotegerin ligand and inhibition of osteoprotegerin production by glucocorticoids in human osteoblastic lineage cells: potential paracrine mechanisms of glucocorticoid-induced osteoporosis. Endocrinology 1999; 140:4382–9.

Johnston CC, Miller JZ, Slemenda CW et al. Calcium supplementation and increases in bone mineral density in children. N Engl J Med 1992; 327:82–7.

Kanis JA, Burlet N, Cooper C et al. European guidance for the diagnosis and management of osteoporosis in postmenopausal women. Osteoporos Int 2008; 19:399–428.

Karasik D, Ferrari SL. Contribution of gender-specific genetic factors to osteoporosis risk. Ann Hum Genet 2008; 72:696–714.

Kearns AE, Khosla S, Kostenuik PJ. Receptor activator of nuclear factor kappa B ligand and osteoprotegerin regulation of bone remodeling in health and disease. Endocr Rev 2008; 29:155–92.

Khosla S. Estrogen and the death of osteoclasts: a fascinating story. BoneKey 2007; 4:267–72.

Khosla S, Riggs BL, Atkinson EJ et al. Effects of sex and age on bone microstructure at the ultradistal radius: a population-based noninvasive in vivo assessment. J Bone Miner Res 2006; 21:124–31.

Komori T. Regulation of osteoblast differentiation by transcription factors. J Cell Biochem 2006; 99:1233–9.

Lee K, Jessop H, Suswillo R et al. Endocrinology: bone adaptation requires oestrogen receptor-alpha. Nature 2003; 424:389.

Lee WT, Leung SS, Leung DM et al. Bone mineral acquisition in low calcium intake children following the withdrawal of calcium supplement. Acta Paediatr 1997; 86:570–6.

Li X, Ominsky MS, Niu QT et al. Targeted deletion of the sclerostin gene in mice results in increased bone formation and bone strength. J Bone Miner Res 2008; 23:860–9.

Li J, Sarosi I, Cattley et al. Dkk1-mediated inhibition of Wnt signaling in bone results in osteopenia. Bone 2006; 39:754–66.

Lindsay R, Aitken JM, Anderson JB et al. Long-term prevention of postmenopausal osteoporosis by oestrogen: evidence for an increased bone mass after delayed onset of oestrogen treatment. Lancet 1976; 1:1038–41.

Lips P, Hosking D, Lippuner K et al. The prevalence of vitamin D inadequacy amongst women with osteoporosis: an international epidemiological investigation. J Intern Med 2006; 260:245–54.

Manolagas SC. Birth and death of bone cells: basic regulatory mechanisms and implications for the pathogenesis and treatment of osteoporosis. Endocr Rev 2000; 21:115–37.

Marcus R. The nature of osteoporosis. In: Osteoporosis. Edited by R Marcus, D

Feldman, J Kelsey. San Diego: Academic Press, 1996; 647–59.

McGuigan FEA, Ralston SH. Genetic susceptibility to osteoporosis. In: Nutritional Aspects of Bone Health. Edited by SA New, JP Bonjour. Cambridge: Royal Society of Chemistry, 2003; 37–63.

Murshed M, Harmey D, Millan JL et al. Unique coexpression in osteoblasts of broadly expressed genes accounts for the spatial restriction of ECM mineralization to bone. Genes Dev 2005; 19:1093–104.

Nakamura T, Imai Y, Matsumoto T et al. Estrogen prevents bone loss via estrogen receptor alpha and induction of Fas ligand in osteoclasts. Cell 2007; 130:811–23.

NIH Consensus Development Panel on Osteoporosis Prevention, Diagnosis, and Therapy. Osteoporosis prevention, diagnosis, and therapy. JAMA 2001; 285:785–95.

Parfitt AM. Targeted and nontargeted bone remodeling: relationship to basic multicellular unit origination and progression. Bone 2002; 30:5–7.

Pei L, Tontonoz P. Fat's loss is bone's gain. J Clin Invest 2004; 113:805–6.

Prince RL, Smith M, Dick IM et al. Prevention of postmenopausal osteoporosis: a comparative study of exercise, calcium supplementation, and hormone-replacement therapy. N Engl J Med 1991; 325:1189–95.

Quigley MET, Martin PL, Burnier AM et al. Estrogen therapy arrests bone loss in elderly women. Am J Obstet Gynecol 1987; 156:1516–23.

Ralston SH. Genetic control of susceptibility to osteoporosis. J Clin Endocrinol Metab 2002; 87:2460–6.

Rauch F, Travers R, Glorieux FH. Cellular activity on the seven surfaces of iliac bone: a histomorphometric study in children and adolescents. J Bone Miner Res 2006; 21:513–9.

Recker R, Lappe J, Davies KM et al. Bone remodeling increases substantially in the years after menopause and remains increased in older osteoporosis patients. J Bone Miner Res 2004; 19:1628–33.

Riggs BL, Khosla S, Melton LJ 3rd. A unitary model for involutional osteoporosis: estrogen deficiency causes both type I and type II osteoporosis in postmenopausal women and contributes to bone loss in aging men. J Bone Miner Res 1998; 13:763–73.

Riggs BL, Khosla S, Melton LJ 3rd et al. Sex steroids and the construction and conservation of the adult skeleton. Endocr Rev 2002; 23:279-302.

Rizzoli R, Ammann P, Chevalley T et al. Protein intake and bone disorders in the elderly. Joint Bone Spine 2001; 68:383–92.

Rizzoli R, Bonjour, J-P. Dietary Protein and Bone Health. J Bone Miner Res 2004; 19:527.

Rodan S, Duong T, Cathepsin K. A new molecular target for osteoporosis. BoneKey 2008; 5:16–24.

Roy D, Swarbrick C, King Y et al. Differences in peak bone mass in women of European and South Asian origin can be explained by differences in body size. Osteoporos Int 2005 (In press).

Schurch MA, Rizzoli R, Slosman D et al. Protein supplements increase serum insulin-like growth factor-I levels and attenuate proximal femur bone loss in patients with recent hip fracture. A randomized, double-blind, placebo-controlled trial. Ann Intern Med 1998; 128:801–9.

Seeman E. Pathogenesis of bone fragility in women and men. Lancet 2002; 359:1841–50.

Seeman E, Hopper JL. Genetic and environmental components of the population variance in bone density. Osteoporos Int 1997; 7(Suppl 3):S10–6.

Seeman E, Delmas PD. Bone quality – the material and structural basis of bone strength and fragility. N Engl J Med 2006; 354:2250–61.

Seeman E, Hopper JL, Bach LA et al. Reduced bone mass in daughters of women with osteoporosis. N Engl J Med 1989; 320:554–8.

Seibel MJ, Woitge HW. Basic principles and clinical applications of biochemical markers of bone metabolism: biochemical and technical aspects. J Clin Densitometry 1999; 2:299–322.

Sornay–Rendu E, Munoz F, Duboeuf F et al. The rate of bone loss is associated with an increased risk of fracture in postmenopausal women. The OFELY study. Osteoporos Int 2005; 16(Suppl 3):OC35.

Standring S (Ed) Gray's anatomy – the anatomical basis of clinical practice, 39th edition. Edinburgh: Elsevier, 2004.

Steingrimsdottir L, Gunnarsson O, Indridason OS et al. Relationship between serum parathyroid hormone levels, vitamin D sufficiency, and calcium intake. JAMA 2005; 294:2336–41.

Styrkarsdottir U, Cazier J, Konng A et al. Linkage of osteoporosis to chromosome 20p12 and association to BMP2. PloS Biology 2003; 1:1–10.

Teitelbaum SL, Ross FP. Genetic regulation of osteoclast development and function. Nat Rev Genet 2003; 4:638–49.

Theintz G, Buchs B, Rizzoli R et al. Longitudinal monitoring of bone mass accumulation in healthy adolescents: evidence for a marked reduction after 16 years of age at the levels of lumbar spine and femoral neck in female subjects. J Clin Endocrinol Metab 1992; 75:1060–5.

Torgerson DJ, Campbell MK, Thomas RE et al. Prediction of perimenopausal fractures by bone mineral density and other risk factors. J Bone Miner Res 1996; 11:293–7.

Vanderschueren D, Bouillon R. Androgens and bone. Calcif Tissue Int 1995; 56:341–346.

van Meurs JB, Trikalinos T, Ralston SH et al. Large-scale analysis of association between polymorphisms in the LRP-5 and -6 genes and osteoporosis: The GENOMOS Study. JAMA 2008; 299:1277–90.

Weitzmann MN, Pacifici R. The role of T lymphocytes in bone metabolism. Immunol Rev 2005; 208:154–68.

Wiren KM, Orwell ES. Skeletal biology of androgens. In: Osteopenia. Edited by R Marcus, D Feldman and J Kelsey. San Diego: Academic Press, 2001;339–359.

Yadav VK, Ryu JH, Suda N et al. Lrp5 controls bone formation by inhibiting serotonin synthesis in the duodenum. Cell 2008; 135:825–37.

Yang X, Karsenty G. Transcription factors in bone: developmental and pathological aspects. Trends Mol Med 2002; 8:340–5.

Chapter 2

Epidemiology and diagnosis of postmenopausal osteoporosis

Juliet Compston and Harry Genant

Prevalence of postmenopausal osteoporosis and the different fractures

Postmenopausal osteoporosis is a common, debilitating disease. The lifetime risk of any fracture occurring in women from the age of 50 years is more than 40% (Figure 2.1) [Kanis et al. 2000]. The lifetime risk of a hip fracture in women is greater than the combined lifetime risks of breast, endometrial, and ovarian cancers. Postmenopausal osteoporosis is also likely to become more common in the decades ahead as the life expectancy of the population increases. The personal and economic burden of postmenopausal osteoporosis results from osteoporotic fractures, which are a significant public health problem, resulting in substantial morbidity and mortality. In the US alone, it has been estimated that around 2 million osteoporotic fractures occur each year. In Europe, it is estimated that more than 30% of women aged 50 years or older have osteoporosis as defined by the World Health Organization (WHO) criteria, with lifetime fracture incidence rates in these women of 14%, 11%, and 13% for hip, vertebral, and distal forearm, respectively [Dennison & Cooper, 2000]. The number of osteoporotic fractures in Europe in 2000 was estimated at 3.79 million [Kanis & Johnell, 2005]. Osteoporosis can develop undetected until a fracture occurs. Any bone can be affected, but fractures of the hip and spine are of special concern; hip fractures because they nearly always result in hospitalization and major surgery, leading to impaired mobility that can be prolonged or permanent, and may even result in death, while vertebral fractures can lead to loss of height, severe back pain and deformity and are also associated with increased mortality.

Risk factors

As in many diseases, several risk factors can be identified in osteoporosis. The identification of risk factors for fracture has been widely used in case finding strategies. Areal bone mineral density (BMD) measured at the lumbar spine and hip, as we will see later in this chapter, is used in the diagnosis of osteoporosis. Low bone mass as measured by BMD is a major risk factor (Figure 2.2), but other factors can provide information on fracture risk that is independent of BMD. These include age, low body mass index, previous fracture, a family history of hip fracture, glucocorticoid therapy, alcohol abuse, tobacco use and rheumatoid arthritis (Figures 2.3–2.8). Increasing age is a significant risk factor, and the incidence of osteoporosis increases with age in both men and women (Figure 2.9). Female gender is also significant, since the virtual withdrawal of estrogen at the menopause hastens the age-related decline in bone mass (Figure 2.10). A personal history of osteoporotic fracture is also an important risk factor (Figure 2.11–2.12). It has been shown that in women who developed a vertebral fracture, the incidence of an additional fracture within the next year was 19.2% [Lindsay et al. 2001]. History of fracture in a patient's mother or maternal grandmother is also associated with an increased risk of fracture [Torgerson et al. 1996; Siris et al. 2001]. In one study, it was found that a maternal history of hip fracture doubled the risk of hip fracture (relative risk [95% confidence interval] 2.0 [1.4–2.9]) [Cummings et al. 1995]. Risk factors that are BMD-dependent include early menopause, either occurring naturally or because of surgery, which increases the risk of developing osteoporosis. Women who stop menstruating before menopause because of conditions such as anorexia nervosa, or because of excessive exercise, can lose bone, leading to the development of osteoporosis. Finally, various lifestyle factors also increase the risk of osteoporosis, including a life-long low calcium intake, a lack of exercise and chronic immobility. Drugs that have been associated with increased risk of osteoporosis include glucocorticoids, aromatase inhibitors, androgen deprivation therapy, proton pump inhibitors, selective serotonin reuptake inhibitors and thiazolidinediones [Compston et al. 2008].

Risk factors that predict fracture independently of bone mineral density are used in the WHO supported algorithm, FRAX® [www.shef.ac.uk/FRAX]. FRAX® (Figure 2.13) can be used with or without bone mineral density to estimate the 10-year probability of a major osteoporotic fracture (hip, spine, wrist, and humerus) or of hip fracture alone [Kanis et al. 2008].

There are significant racial differences in the incidence of osteoporosis (Figure 2.14), and in the incidence of osteoporotic fracture. In the US, postmenopausal osteoporosis has repeatedly been noted to be more common in white non-Hispanic women and in Asian women than it is in Hispanic women and African-American women [National Osteoporosis Foundation, 1997]. This may be explained by the higher peak bone mass achieved before the menopause in African-American women. Asian women may be at an increased risk of osteoporotic fracture because of their lower body weight, this being an independent risk factor for osteoporosis.

Vertebral deformity and fracture

Although not the highest contributors to the direct economic costs of osteoporosis, vertebral fractures are the most common type of osteoporotic fracture. Only approximately one out of three osteoporotic vertebral fractures is diagnosed in clinical practice because the diagnosis almost always depends on the patient reporting back pain that is severe enough for a radiograph to be ordered, and fewer than 10% necessitate hospital admission [Papaioannou et al. 2002]. The prevalence of radiographic vertebral deformity increases with age; for example, in Europe the prevalence rises from 11.5% in women aged 50–54 years to 34.8% in women aged 75–79 [O'Neill et al. 1996]. Overall, up to 26% of postmenopausal women have been reported as having a vertebral deformity [Lau, 2001]. Vertebral fractures most commonly occur at the junction of the thoracic and lumbar spines, and in the mid-thoracic area (Figure 2.15) [Papaioannou et al. 2002], and are associated with back pain, kyphosis, and excess mortality, possibly through coexisting frailty.

Hip fracture

Hip fractures are a major cause of morbidity and mortality in the elderly (Figures 2.16–2.19). Their incidence increases exponentially with age, beginning to rise only very slowly at the time of menopause, but starting to increase dramatically around the age of 70 years (Figure 2.20). The number of hip fractures occurring worldwide is expected to increase to 6.26 million by 2050 [Cummings & Melton, 2002], marking an almost fourfold increase in hip fractures since 1990. In 2000, the number of hip fractures was estimated to be 890,000 in Europe alone [Kanis & Johnell, 2005].

Other types of fracture

The other type of fracture most commonly cited as being osteoporotic is of the distal forearm, either a Colles' fracture (Figure 2.21) or a Smith's fracture. Unlike vertebral and hip fractures, the incidence of forearm fractures increases slowly in the early years after the menopause, but then levels out. It has been suggested that this may be because younger women are more likely to break their fall on an outstretched arm whereas older women, who tend to have a slower gait and poorer neuromuscular coordination, are more likely to fall sideways or backwards, landing on their hip [Nevitt & Cummings, 1993] (Figure 2.22). It is more difficult to determine whether fractures at other sites are related to osteoporosis. Nevertheless, the incidence of other fractures in women (excluding fractures of the face, skull, and ribs) has been shown to slightly more than double with age between 55 and 80 years [De Laet & Pols, 2000], which strongly suggests that at least some of these other fractures are the result of osteoporosis.

Diagnosis of osteoporosis

History and physical examination

History and physical examination alone are not sufficient to diagnose osteoporosis. They are, however, important components of the screening process and can identify risk factors that are potentially amenable to change, and give clues about the presence of established osteoporosis that may warrant further investigation. Evaluation of calcium intake in the diet, using a diet questionnaire, is a commonly used method of screening for risk. Historically, osteoporosis is clinically silent and diagnosis was, therefore, generally not made until the bone had become sufficiently weak to fracture. Clearly this is less than ideal, since treatments are available to prevent osteoporosis or slow its development. Osteoporosis is known to be associated with low bone mass and, on that basis, various diagnostic and screening tests have been devised to assess BMD. The WHO has produced classification and diagnostic guidelines for osteoporosis, based on BMD measurements [World Health Organization, 1994]. Although osteoporosis that is sufficiently advanced can be visualized on plain radiographs, BMD must be decreased by approximately 50% before this is possible. Therefore, an apparently normal appearance on plain radiographs cannot exclude osteoporosis [Garton et al. 1994]. Moreover, significant observer variation in the assessment of bone density using plain radiographs has been reported.

Bone mineral density measurement

BMD measurement remains the gold standard for the diagnosis of osteoporosis. A patient's BMD is often expressed by its relationship to two norms:
- the expected BMD for 'young normal' adults of the same sex (T-score);
- the expected BMD for the patient's age and sex (Z-score).

The difference between the patient's score and the norm is expressed in terms of standard deviations (SD) above or below the mean. In broad terms, 1 SD represents 10–20% of the bone density value. In the normal ageing population, T-scores decline in parallel with the steady drop in bone mass that occurs with ageing. Osteoporosis is defined as a BMD T-score of less than or equal to –2.5, and osteopenia (Figure 2.23) as a T-score between –1 and –2.5 (Figure 2.24). It should be noted that these criteria apply only to measurements obtained by dual-X-ray absorptiometry (DXA). The techniques for measuring bone may be broadly divided into those that measure the central skeleton, and those that measure some part of the peripheral skeleton. There is only moderate correlation between BMD at various sites in the body, and BMD at a specific site is the best predictor of the probability of fracture at that site [Marshall et al. 1996].

Dual-X-ray absorptiometry

BMD of the central skeleton is normally measured using DXA, which is currently the most effective way of estimating postmenopausal fracture risk, certainly in Caucasian women. DXA is used to measure the bone mineral content of the entire skeleton, and at specific sites that are vulnerable to fracture. The bone mineral content can be used to derive the BMD, by measuring the mineral content at a specific site and dividing it by the area measured (Figure 2.25). Although this technique provides a two-dimensional areal value rather than a volumetric density, with the size of the bone affecting the apparent density, DXA can help determine skeletal strength, as this is influenced by the bone size. The best location for the use of DXA to measure BMD is at the hip. Diagnosis of osteoporosis using BMD findings from DXA relies on the use of population-based reference range databases. Reference ranges of BMD are available for determining osteoporosis in European women using measurements from Hologic machines, and in American women as proposed by the WHO and International Osteoporosis Foundation. Similar databases are being established for Asian and African women. The use of BMD has shown that for elderly women with very low BMD (T-score < –3.5) there is a twofold higher risk of hip fracture than the average risk for women of the same age [Dargent-Molina et al. 2002]. This study also showed that the use of femoral neck BMD, together with clinical risk factors, was able to identify another subset of women who were at double the average risk of fracture; this, therefore, increases the efficiency of selective BMD screening.

The preferred sites for DXA measurement are the lumbar spine (L1–L4) (Figure 2.26) and hip (Figure 2.27), with the latter being preferred in older women and men (approximately >65 years) when degenerative changes (eg, osteophytes, sclerosis, aortic calcification) interfere more significantly with

BMD measurement in the spine. Diagnosis of osteoporosis using DXA-derived BMD relies on the use of population-based reference range databases. By comparison of BMD results to these references ranges, T-scores or age- and ethnicity-matched Z-scores can be computed. Z-scores are recommended in premenopausal women and men under the age of 50 years while T-scores, found by comparing BMD with young normal values for Caucasians, are often used in older patients. Z- and T-scores can be used to diagnose osteoporosis using WHO standards or they can be used as inputs along with other risk factors in statistical models to estimate the 10-year absolute fracture risk. Reference ranges are available for the lumbar spine from each DXA manufacturer while reference data for the hip from the US based NHANES III study have become the recognized standard around the world. Similar databases are being established for Asian men and women [Cui et al. 2008; Fujiwara et al. 2008].

Quantitative ultrasound and quantitative computed tomography

At present, quantitative ultrasound can be used to predict fracture risk, but it cannot be used for the diagnosis of osteoporosis, or for monitoring the effects of treatment, because the results of quantitative ultrasound (Figure 2.28) do not correlate well with BMD measurements and there are no population based standards [Glüer & Hans, 1999]. Quantitative computed tomography is used extensively in clinical research, as it gives additional compartment specific volumetric BMD information; however, it uses higher radiation exposure and is less accessible than DXA. It is, nevertheless, the best noninvasive method for separately measuring trabecular and cortical volumetric density (Figure 2.29) [Genant et al. 1982; 1996].

Radiological assessment of vertebral fractures

Semiquantitative methods

A number of semiquantitative (SQ) methods for assessing vertebral fractures have been developed, but only the Genant SQ method (Figure 2.30), which has been extensively used in clinical drug trials and epidemiological studies, will be described here [Genant et al. 1993; Genant & Jergas, 2003]. The correct qualitative classification of a vertebral deformity can be achieved only through visual inspection, and interpretation of the radiograph. In the Genant method, the severity of the fracture is assessed solely by visual determination, which involves determining the extent of the vertebral height reduction and morphological changes, and differentiating the fracture from other non-fracture deformities. Grades are assigned to each vertebra based on the approximate degree of height reduction. This method does not link the type of deformity with the grading of the fracture. When using this method the thoracic and lumbar vertebrae from T4 to L4 are graded using the following definitions:

- grade 0 is normal
- grade 0.5 is 'borderline', where the vertebra shows some deformation, but this is not clearly assignable to grade 1 fractures
- grade 1 is mildly deformed, with an approximate 20–25% reduction in anterior, middle and/or posterior height and a 10–20% reduction in the projected vertebral area
- grade 2 is moderately deformed, with an approximate 25–40% reduction in anterior, middle and/or posterior height and 20–40% reduction in the projected vertebral area
- grade 3 is severely deformed, with an approximate 40% or more reduction in anterior, middle and/or posterior height and the projected vertebral area.

In addition, careful attention should be paid to alterations in the shape and configuration of the vertebrae relative to adjacent vertebrae and expected normal appearances, which can add a strong qualitative, sometimes subjective, aspect to the interpretation. Buckling or bowing of the vertebral endplates or cortices provides strong supportive evidence of a vertebral fracture [Jiang et al. 2007]. A spinal deformity index (SDI) can be calculated from these results by adding together all of the grades assigned to the T4–L4 vertebrae as a measure of total spinal burden of fracture [Genant et al. 2005]. One advantage of this SQ method is that by assessing the severity of the deformation, as a reduction of vertebral height, refractures of preexisting vertebral fractures can be assessed within the range of grading. When assessing incident vertebral fractures, it is necessary to examine serial radiographs from the patient to provide a thorough and reliable analysis of all new fractures.

Quantitative methods

Bone scintigraphy scans sometimes reveal a recent vertebral fracture that cannot be seen on plain radiography. All current quantitative morphometric methods for determining vertebral dimensions use electronic digitizing procedures. These methods usually use six points to derive the anterior height (ha), central (middle or mid-vertebral) height (hm) and posterior height (hp) (Figure 2.25). The most widely used calculated parameters are wedge ratio (ha/hp), biconcave ratio (hm/hp) and compression ratio ($ha/hp+1$), where 1 indicates the vertebral body above or below) [Genant & Jergas, 2003]. Various thresholds have been set for these measurements and there are clear differences found between the assessments for prevalent and incident vertebral fractures, owing to the way in which normative vertebral dimensions and vertebral deformities are defined. Therefore, adjustments have to be performed to take into account the normal anatomical shape of the vertebral body, as it is not a perfect rectangle. It is known that the ha of the vertebral body is smaller than the hp in the midthoracic vertebral bodies, is equal to the hp in the thoracolumbar region, and is greater than the hp in the lower lumbar levels, while lumbar vertebral bodies are generally bigger than thoracic vertebral bodies. Magnetic resonance imaging can be used to look for other pathology in a fractured vertebra, and it may reveal bone marrow edema, a sign of a recent fracture [Ross, 1997; Papaioannou et al. 2002] (Figure 2.31).

Economic cost of fractures

Osteoporotic fractures result in a significant economic cost (Figure 2.32). In Europe, the total direct costs of osteoporotic fractures in 2000 were estimated at 31.7 billion euros and, with an aging population, this is expected to increase to 76.7 billion euros by 2050 [Kanis & Johnell, 2005]. In the US, healthcare expenditure attributable to osteoporotic fractures in 2005 was estimated at $US16.9 billion with a projected cost of $US25.3 billion by 2025. Hip fractures accounted for approximately 63% of the total healthcare expenditure attributed to osteoporotic fractures [Ray et al. 1997].

Effect of fractures on independence, quality of life, and mortality

Osteoporosis and the fractures it causes are a major source of morbidity. The sequelae of osteoporotic hip fractures are often severe, and may be devastating (Figure 2.33). Predominantly affecting the very elderly, they result in permanent disability in over 30% of patients, and up to 20% die within one year of their fracture, the majority of deaths occuring within the first six months (Figures 2.34 and 2.35). Hip fractures also lead to a greater risk of functional impairment and institutionalization. One year following a hip fracture, it has been found that 40% of patients are unable to walk independently, 60% cannot carry out at least one activity of daily living, and 80% or more are unable to carry out at least one independent activity of daily living, such as shopping or driving [Cooper, 1997]. In another study the effect of hip fracture was studied in a cohort of 120 community-living individuals over 65 years of age [Marottoli et al. 1992]. Within six months of fracture, 22 of the cohort had died, while 49% could not dress independently (compared with 86% at baseline), 32% could not transfer independently (versus 90%), 15% could not walk across a room independently (versus 75%), 8% could not climb a flight of stairs independently (versus 63%), and 6% could not walk half a mile independently (versus 41%). Vertebral fractures are a major cause of back pain, and loss of height in the elderly. Alterations in the contour of the spine can cause visceral crowding, including decreased lung function [Schlaich et al. 1998]. Vertebral fractures are also associated with increased mortality, with one study finding that women with vertebral fractures have a 16% reduction in expected five-year survival [Cooper et al. 1993].

Remaining lifetime risk of fracture (%) at 50 years of age

Figure 2.1. There is variation between men and women in the risk of fracture at different sites at 50 years of age. In women, the remaining lifetime risk of any fracture at the age of 50 years was 46.4% compared with just 22.4% for men. In women, the risk of hip fracture was the highest, followed by forearm, vertebral, and proximal humerus fractures. In men, the pattern is similar, but there are more vertebral fractures than forearm fractures. Data from Kanis JA, Johnell O, Oden A et al. Long-term risk of osteoporotic fracture in Malmö. Osteoporos Int 2000; 11:669–74.

Fracture site	Women (%)	Men (%)
Forearm	20.8	4.6
Hip	22.9	10.7
Proximal humerus	12.9	4.1
Vertebral	15.1	8.3
Any of these	46.4	22.4

Prevalence of low bone mineral density by age in women

Figure 2.2. The data are from a population-based estimate for Rochester, USA. The graph shows the proportion of women with a bone mineral density (BMD) T-score less than –2 at three sites: lumbar spine, hip, and at one of the spine, hip, or mid-radius. The prevalence of low BMD increases dramatically at approximately 50 years (corresponding with the menopause) and continues to increase thereafter. Adapted from Melton LJ 3rd. How many women have osteoporosis now? J Bone Miner Res 1995; 10:175–7.

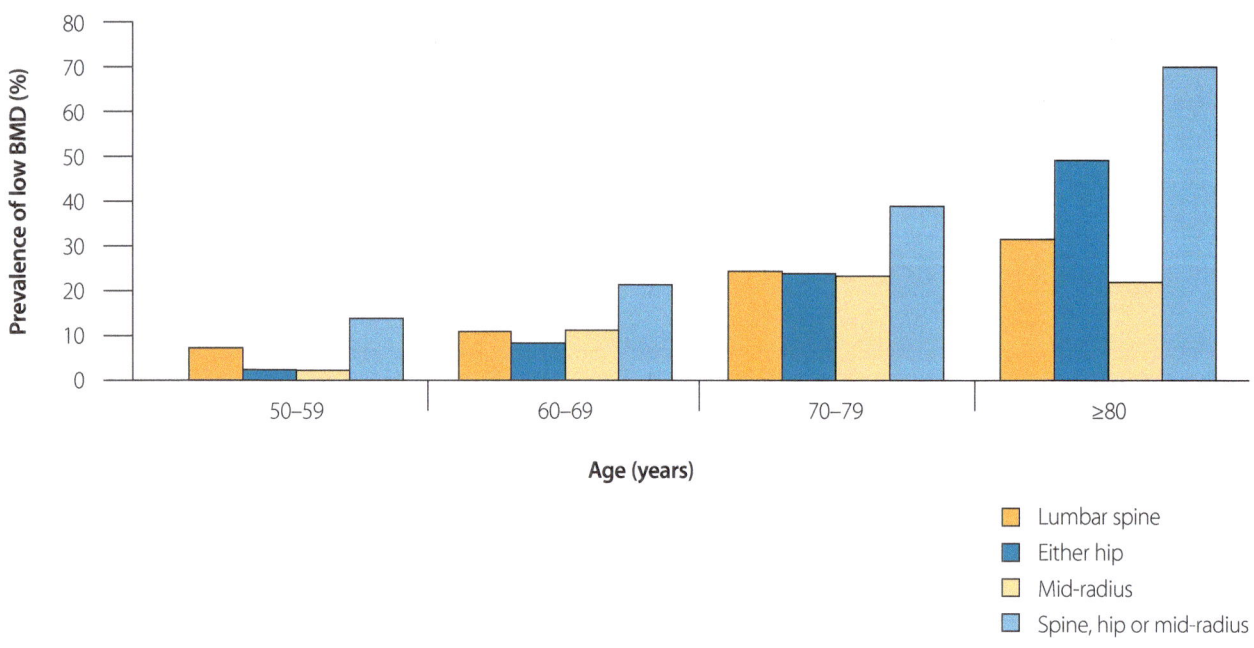

Risk factors for osteoporotic fracture

Figure 2.3. The risk factors shown in the left hand column act, at least in part, independently of bone mineral density (BMD) and hence improve the prediction of fracture risk over the use of BMD measurements alone. With the exception of falls, these are utilized in the FRAX® algorithm, developed by the World Health Organization, for the prediction of fracture risk (see also Figure 2.13). The risk factors in the right hand column increase fracture risk mainly or exclusively through their effect on BMD. Risk factors for falls include environmental hazards, such as poor lighting, loose carpets and uneven paving stones, and intrinsic factors such as neuromuscular disease, poor balance, decreased visual acuity and cardiovascular disease.

BMD independent	BMD dependent
Age	Hypogonadism
Female gender	Immobility
Parental history of hip fracture	Hyperthyroidism
Previous fragility fracture	Gastrointestinal disease
Glucocorticoid therapy	Chronic renal disease
Low body mass index	Chronic liver disease
Alcohol abuse	Type 1 diabetes
Smoking	Organ transplantation
Rheumatoid arthritis	Chronic obstructive pulmonary disease
Falls	Drugs

Risk factors associated with hip fracture from a fall

Figure 2.4. An age- and sex-matched case-control study was conducted to examine the interaction between bone mineral density (BMD) and a number of factors (body mass index, predisposing medical conditions, fall characteristics, functional mobility, and femoral neck BMD) as risk factors for hip fracture risk. The study included 252 community-dwelling elderly patients aged between 65 and 85 years: 127 who fell and sustained a hip fracture (case patients), and 125 who fell, but did not sustain a hip fracture (controls). Multiple logistic regression analysis of the data showed that both sideways fall and direct hip impact were strong and independent risk factors for hip fracture. In the different analysis sets, the effect of risk factors remained the same, and adding or removing femoral neck BMD did not change other risk factors. BMD was, however, significantly correlated with functional mobility and body mass index. These results are similar to a study by Greenspan et al. [1994], which showed that a person who falls sideways is six times more likely to sustain a hip fracture than one who falls in other directions. This study also showed that the risk of hip fracture increased nearly three times for every one standard deviation decrease in femoral BMD compared with the mean BMD, and approximately doubled for each standard deviation decrease in body mass index. These findings indicate that BMD measurement does not capture all of the determinants of hip fracture. Adapted from Wei TS, Hu CH, Wang SH et al. Fall characteristics, functional mobility and bone mineral density as risk factors of hip fracture in the community-dwelling ambulatory elderly. Osteoporos Int 2001; 12:1050–5.

Factor	Adjusted odds ratio	95% confidence interval
Direct hip impact	4.9	2.7–8.8
Previous stroke	2.9	1.3–6.3
Sideways fall	2.5	1.6–3.9
Functional mobility	2.0	1.1–3.5
Body mass index	1.8	1.1–2.8
Femoral neck BMD	1.7	1.0–2.8

Average 10-year probability of hip fracture according to age and relative risk

Figure 2.5. The use of risk factors for predicting the likelihood of having a fracture has been examined. The results show the 10-year probability of hip fracture in women according to age and relative risk. The symbols show the effect of risk factors on fracture probability derived from two studies of women aged either 65 years (OFELY), or 80 years (EPIDOS). It should be noted that the data from the OFELY study are derived from information on all fractures. The threshold values used for the risk factors were a T-score <–2.5 for low bone mineral density (BMD), presence of prior fracture and above premenopausal values for type 1 C-telopeptide (CTX) breakdown products, low BMD plus prior fracture, low BMD plus high CTX, prior fracture plus high CTX, and all of the above. The results showed that age is an important determinant of fracture probability, but at any given age the presence of a single risk factor is associated with a doubling of the 10-year probability, and this increases markedly when risk factors are combined. From Johnell O, Oden A, De Laet C et al. Biochemical indices of bone turnover and the assessment of fracture probability. Osteoporos Int 2002; 13:523–6.

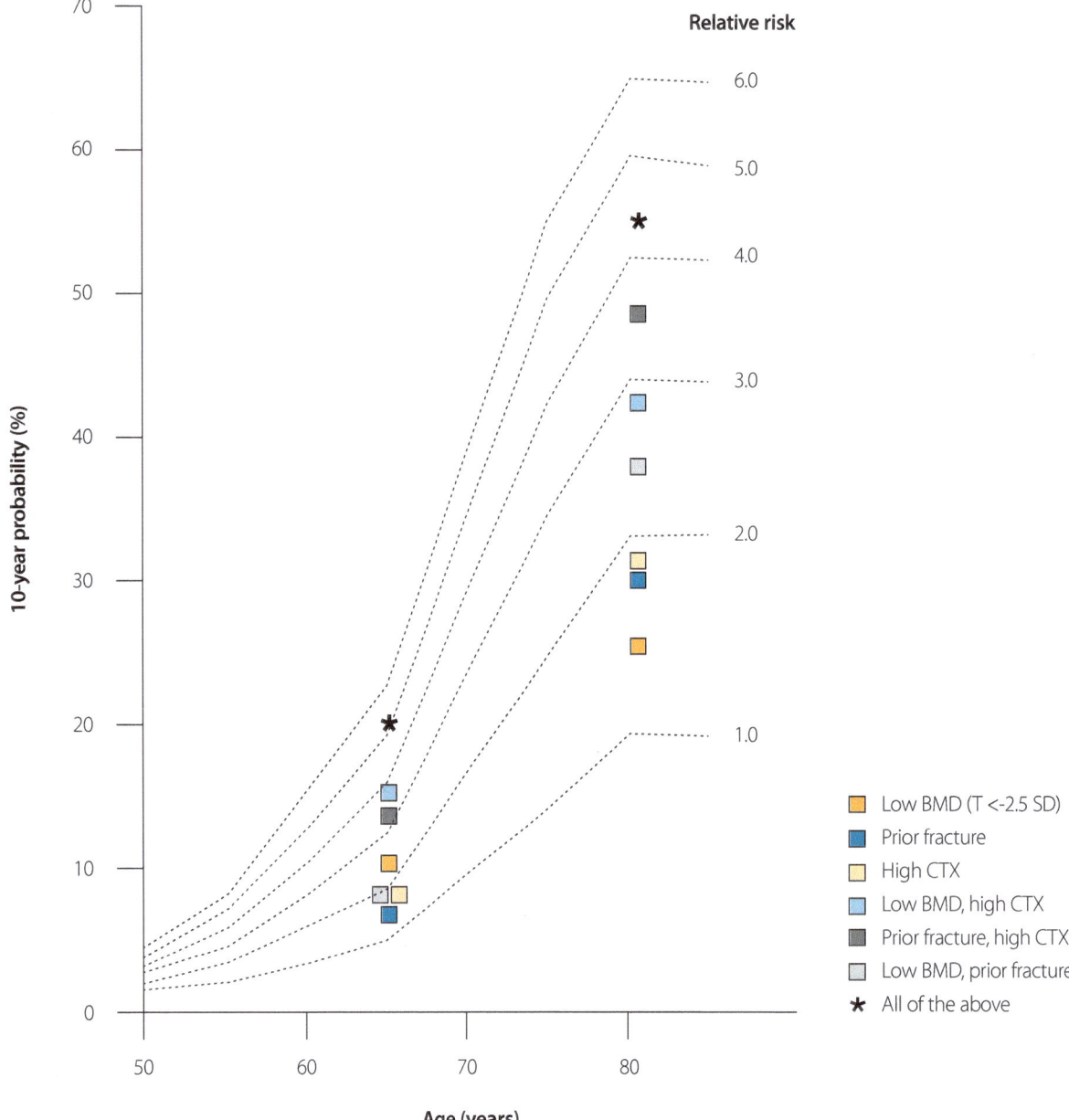

Effect of excessive alcohol intake on fracture risk

Figure 2.6. This study looked at the effect of reported alcohol intake on the risk of any fracture, any osteoporotic fracture and hip fracture alone in over 16,000 patients from three prospective study cohorts. No significant increase in risk is observed at intakes of 2 units of alcohol or less daily. Above this threshold alcohol intake was associated with an increased risk of any fracture (risk ratio [RR] = 1.23; 95% CI, 1.06–1.43), any osteoporotic fracture (RR =1.38; 95% CI, 1.16–1.65), or hip fracture (RR =1.68; 95% CI, 1.19–2.39). There was no significant interaction with age, bone mineral density (BMD) or evidence of a different threshold for effect by gender. This figure shows intake divided into more than 2, more than 3 and more than 4 units of alcohol daily (vs those who took less). In both men and women risk ratios were increased with higher categories of intake and were significantly increased in both sexes with intakes of more than 2 units daily. From Kanis J, Johansson H, Johnell O et al. Alcohol intake as a risk factor for fracture. Osteoporosis Int 2005a; 16:7370–42.

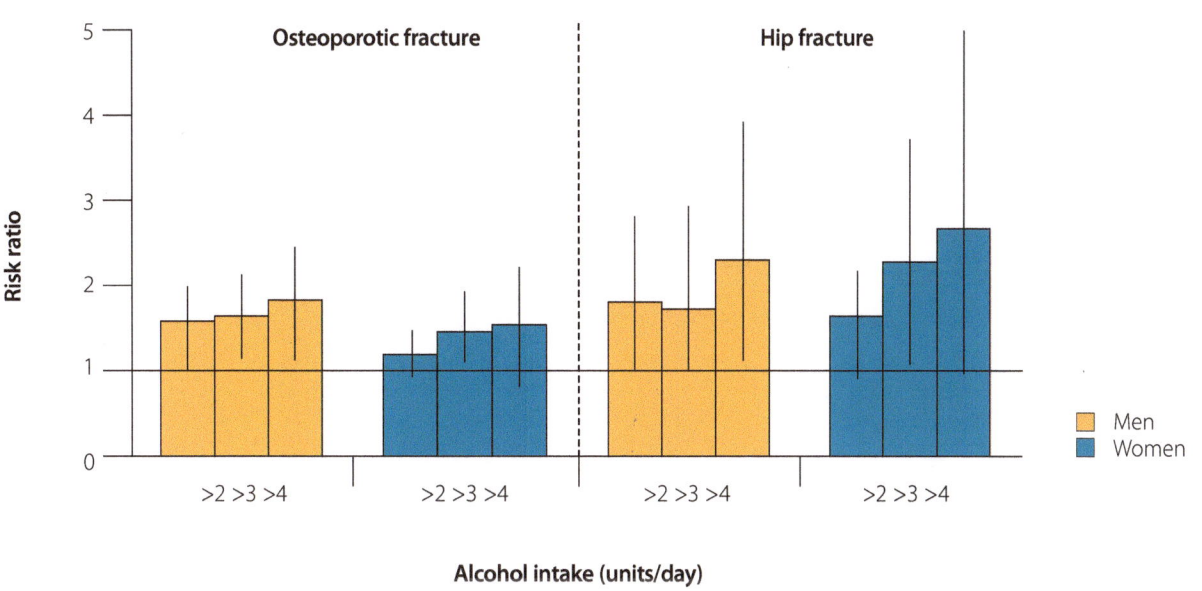

Effect of excessive cigarette smoking on fracture risk

Figure 2.7. Smoking is also considered a risk factor for fracture. The figure below is from a study that examined 59,232 men and women from 10 prospective cohorts. Current smoking was associated with a significantly increased risk of any fracture compared with nonsmokers (risk ratio [RR] =1.25; 95% CI, 1.15–1.36). RR was adjusted marginally downward when bone mineral density (BMD) was taken into account, but it remained significantly increased (RR =1.13). The highest risk was observed for hip fracture (RR =1.84; 95% CI, 1.52–2.22). A smoking history was associated with a significantly increased risk of fracture compared with individuals with no smoking history, but the risk ratios were lower than for current smoking. A history of smoking results in fracture risk that is substantially greater than that explained by measurement of BMD. Data from Kanis J, Johnell O, Oden A. Smoking and fracture risk: a meta-analysis. Osteoporos Int 2005b; 16:155–62.

Risk of fracture associated with current smoking	Type of fracture		
	Any	Osteoporotic	Hip
Risk ratio	1.25	1.29	1.84
Risk ratio adjusted for BMD	1.13	1.13	1.60

10-year probability of a major osteoporotic fracture in men and women aged 65 years according to T-score and clinical risk factors

Figure 2.8. 10-year probability of a major osteoporotic fracture in men and women aged 65 years according to T-score and clinical risk factors. Body mass index is set at 25 kg/m². The 10-year probability of a major osteoporotic fracture (hip, spine, wrist or humerus) is plotted against femoral neck T-score for men (top) and women (bottom) aged 65 years with body mass index of 25 kg/m². The graphs show how risk factors such as prior fracture, glucocorticoid therapy and family history increase the fracture risk independently of bone mineral density. The effect of these clinical risk factors on fracture risk is additive; thus glucocorticoid therapy in combination with prior fracture produces a greater fracture probability than prior fracture alone, and when a family history of fracture is added the fracture probability rises further. From Kanis A, Johnell O, Oden A et al. FRAX™ and the assessment of fracture probability in men and women from the UK. Osteoporos Int 2008a; 19:385–97.

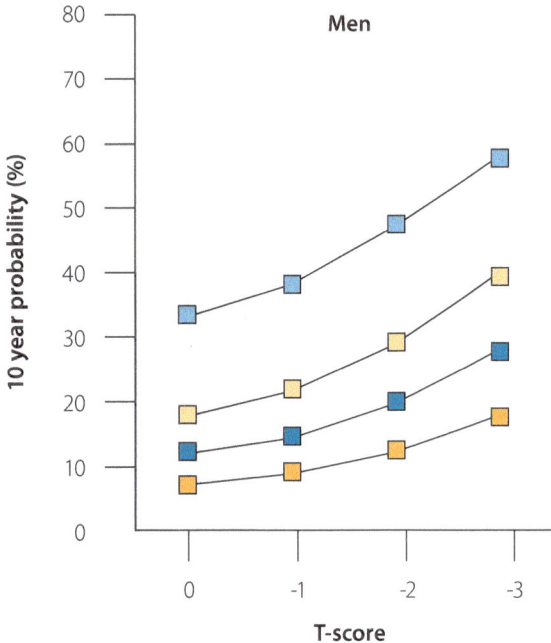

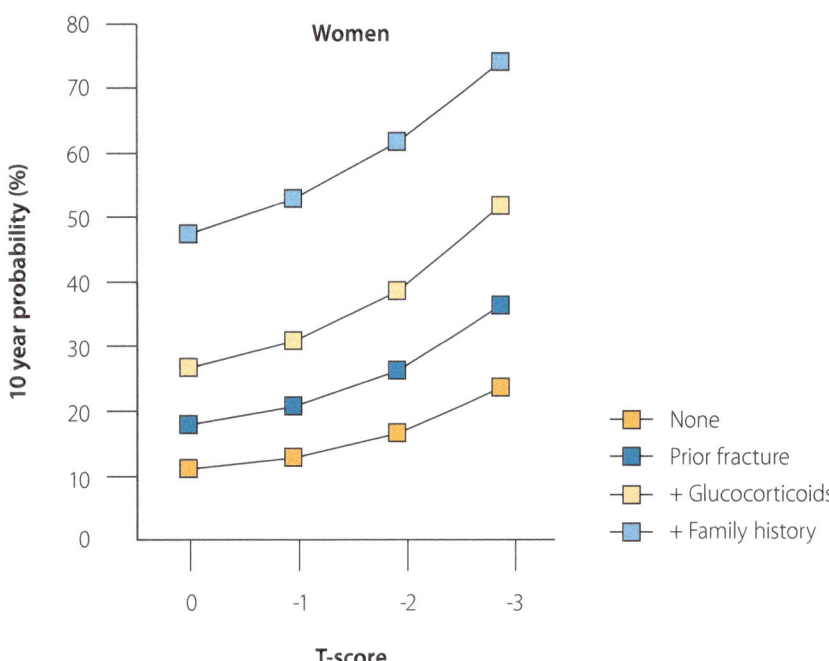

Age-related fractures

Figure 2.9. The incidence of fractures increases with age after the menopause in women and about 10 years later in men. The incidence in hip fracture increases markedly in both women and men in old age owing, in part, to the increased incidence of falls in the elderly and the greater likelihood that an elderly person will fall on his or her hip. Conversely, the risk of wrist fracture in women tends to level out with age, possibly because an older person is less likely to fall onto the outstretched arm. The incidence of osteoporotic fractures, which are largely unrelated to trauma, also rises sharply with age in later life. Adapted from Cooper C, Melton LJ III. Epidemiology of osteoporosis. Trends Endocrinol Metab 1992; 3:224–9.

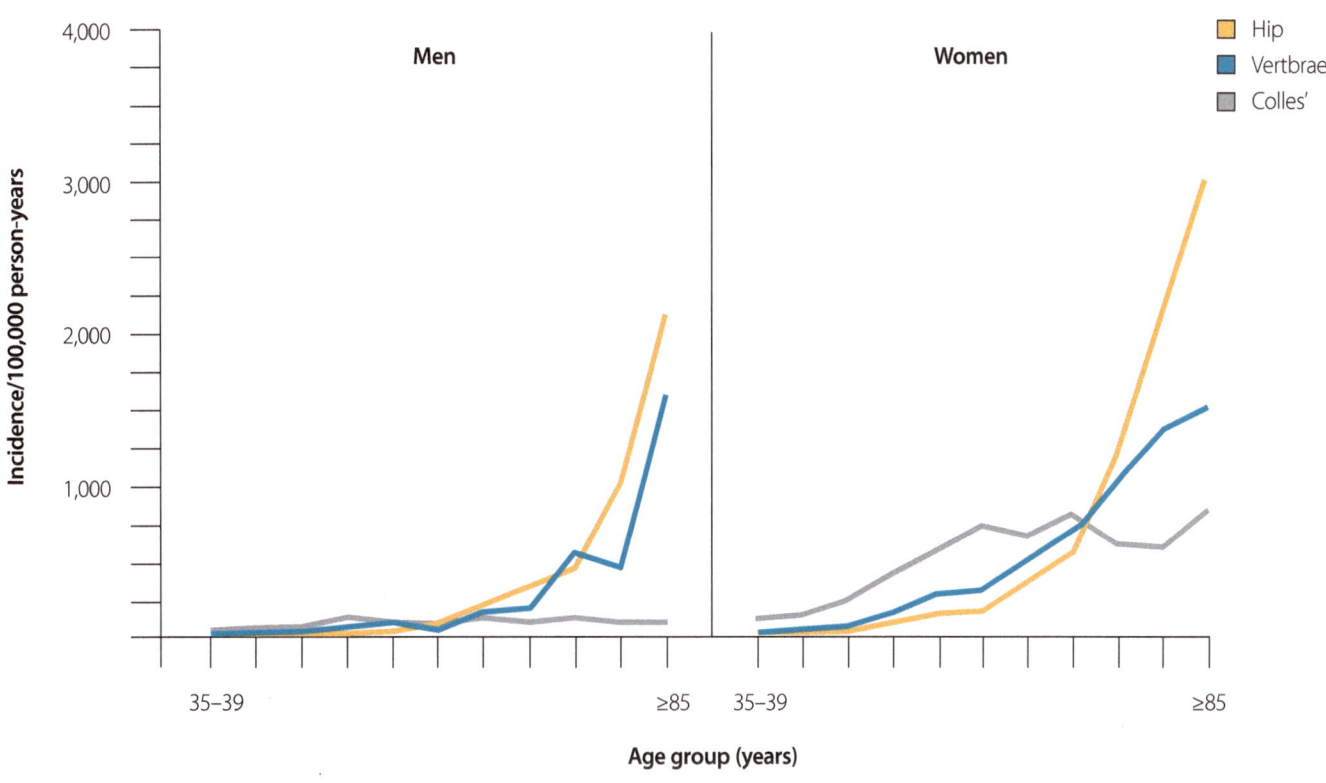

Lifetime changes in bone mass

Figure 2.10. Bone mineral density (BMD) increases throughout childhood, adolescence, and early adulthood, reaching peak levels by the early 20s. Peak bone mass is higher in women than in men. Bone loss in both sexes probably starts during the fourth decade of life and continues throughout life thereafter. The onset of the menopause brings with it a virtually complete withdrawal of circulating estrogen, causing a noticeable increase in the rate of loss of bone mass in women. This menopause-related bone loss typically lasts approximately 10 years, after which bone loss continues, but at a slower rate. In men there is no accelerated phase of bone loss and the rate of bone loss is similar to that seen in older postmenopausal women. The risk of fractures increases with decreasing BMD.

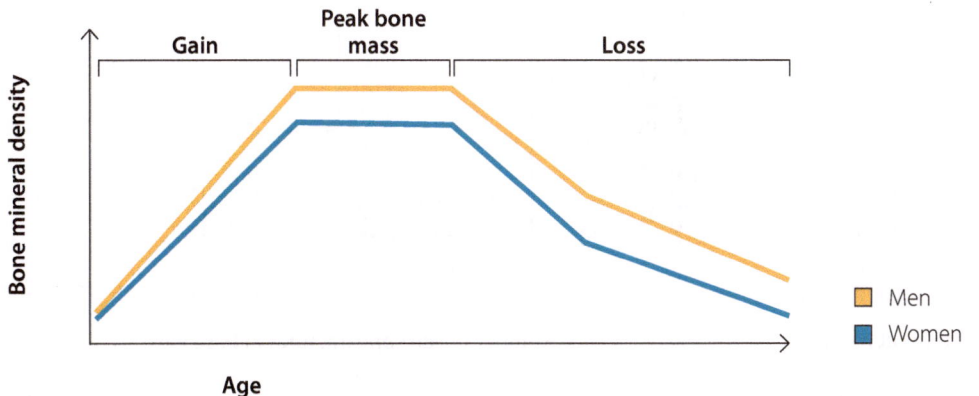

Relationship between prior and subsequent fractures

Figure 2.11. The data are taken from a number of different studies that showed associations between various prior fractures and subsequent fractures. Nine studies found an association between prior wrist fractures and subsequent fracture, with only one of the studies limited to postmenopausal women, and the remainder being in women 45 years or older, or in both men and women. Fifteen studies showed an association between prior vertebral fracture and subsequent fractures, with seven based on prior clinical vertebral fractures, and the rest based on prior morphometric fractures identified at baseline using radiographs. Most of these studies were in women who were postmenopausal when the fractures were diagnosed, the others were in men and women, and in one instance in men only. Six studies found an association between prior hip fracture and subsequent fracture; the majority involved women only, one was in men only, and one in men and women. Nineteen studies showed an association between fracture at any site and subsequent fracture in a mixture of patient groups. It was found that although the magnitude varied, having a history of prior fracture at any site is an important risk factor for subsequent fractures. *The results are pooled estimates of any subsequent fracture at the wrist, vertebral, all (or non-spine) or hip; [†]other relative risk estimates were reported, but were not included in the pooled estimates because measures of variability were lacking or because estimates were biased owing to differences in follow-up; [‡]excludes prior vertebral fracture predicting subsequent vertebral fracture, because stronger associations were observed. Adapted from Klotzbuecher CM, Ross PD, Landsman PB et al. Patients with prior fractures have an increased risk of future fractures: a summary of the literature and statistical synthesis. J Bone Miner Res 2000; 15:721–39.

Location of prior fracture	Population	Risk of subsequent fracture*
Wrist	Peri/postmenopausal	2.0[†]
	Other	2.6
Vertebral	Peri/postmenopausal	1.9[‡]
	Other	2.3[‡]
Other (all, or specific sites)	Peri/postmenopausal	1.9[†]
	Other	1.7[†]
Hip	Peri/postmenopausal	2.4
	other	1.7

Incidence of vertebral fracture by number of baseline vertebral fractures

Figure 2.12. It has been found that the presence of one or more vertebral fractures at baseline increases the risk of sustaining a subsequent vertebral fracture within the next year by fivefold. The study analyzed data from postmenopausal women included in the placebo arm of four large three-year osteoporosis treatment trials, in whom vertebral fracture status was known at entry. The mean age of these women was 74 years, and they had a mean of 28 years since menopause. **(a)** Results for first year of study, and **(b)** Results for first year after vertebral fracture during study. The incidence is based on Kaplan–Meier estimates of the survival function. CI, confidence interval. Reproduced with permission from Lindsay R, Silverman SL, Cooper C et al. Risk of new vertebral fracture in the year following a fracture. JAMA 2001; 285:320–3.

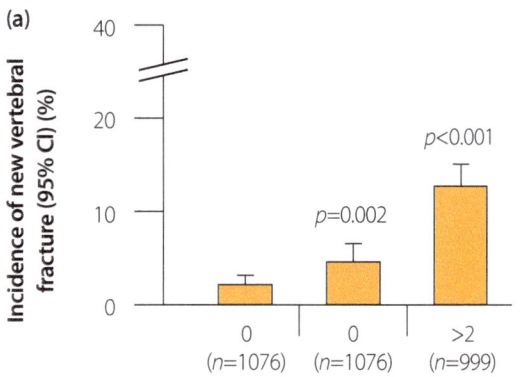

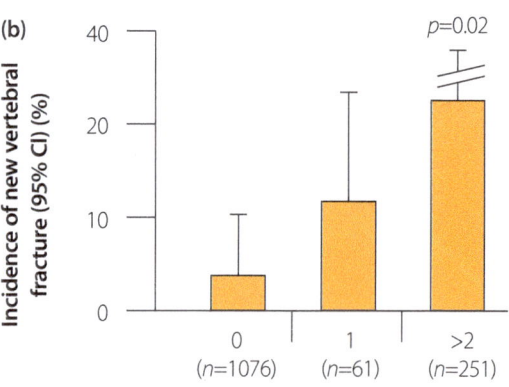

World Health Organization Fracture Risk Assessment Tool

Figure 2.13. The World Health Organization Fracture Risk Assessment tool, FRAX®, can be accessed at www. shef.ac.uk/FRAX. Calculation of fracture probability based on country-specific data is available for China, France, Italy, Japan, Spain, Sweden, Turkey, the UK and the USA. Risk factors are entered as yes /no answers, thus the assessment takes no account of dose–response for risk factors such as previous fracture, glucocorticoid therapy, or smoking. For example, two previous fractures carry a much greater risk of subsequent fracture than one previous fracture, and the effect of glucocorticoids on fracture risk is dose-dependent and this should be taken into account when assessing the individual patient. FRAX® can only be used in postmenopausal women and men aged over 50 years and is not designed to estimate fracture probability in people who have previously received bone protective treatment. The FRAX® tool can be used with or without femoral neck BMD and estimates the 10-year probability of a major osteoporotic fracture (hip, spine, wrist and humerus) or a hip fracture alone. Femoral neck bone mineral density can be entered as either a Z-score or a T-score. Secondary causes of osteoporosis act through reducing bone mineral density and if the 'yes' button is checked femoral neck bone mineral density cannot also be entered. Reproduced with permission from the WHO Collaborating Centre for Metabolic Bone Diseases, University of Sheffield, UK.

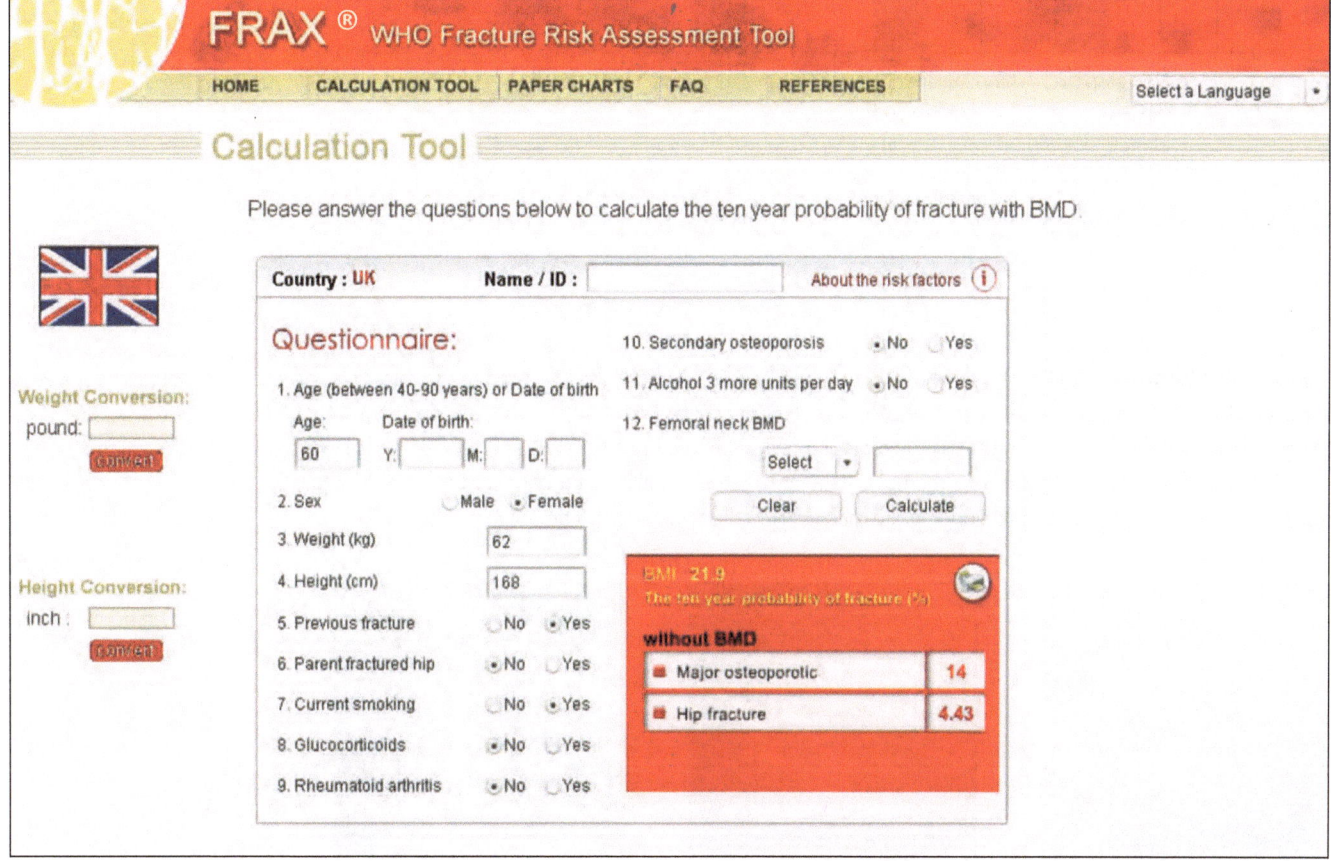

Effect of race on prevalence of osteoporosis or osteopenia in woman aged 50 years or older

Figure 2.14. The percentage of women aged 50 years or older in the USA who have osteoporosis, or osteopenia, was determined in three broad racial groups. Both postmenopausal osteoporosis and osteopenia are more common in non-Hispanic white women and in Asian women than in other racial groups. African-American women have the lowest incidence. The percentages were calculated on the basis of dual-X-ray absorptiometry measurements of femoral neck, trochanteric, and intertrochanteric bone mineral density. Data from National Osteoporosis Foundation. 1996 and 2015 Osteoporosis Prevalence Figures: Stateby-State Report. Washington, DC: National Osteoporosis Foundation; 1997.

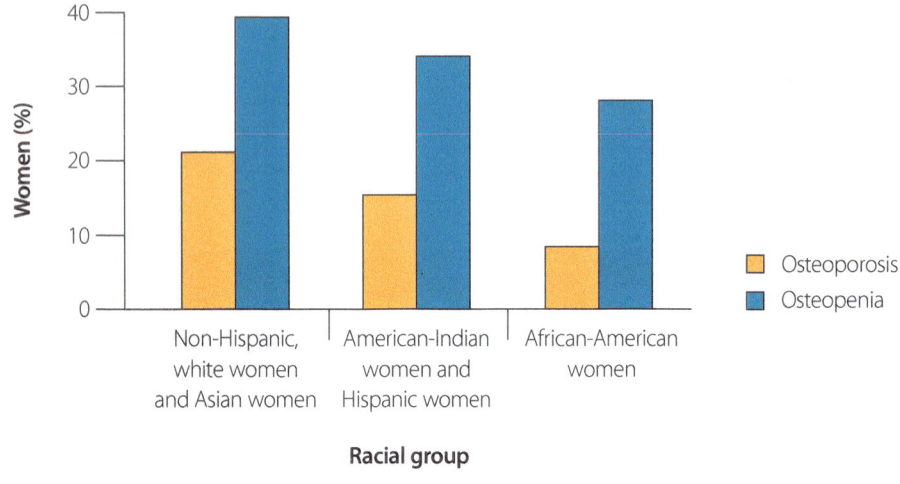

Compression fractures of lumbar vertebrae

Figure 2.15. Progression of vertebral fractures over a 20-year period. The lateral radiograph on the left shows a vertebral fracture of L1. In the middle radiograph, the fracture of L1 has worsened and there is a new fracture at L2. In the radiograph on the right, there are fractures of all the lumbar vertebrae. The collapse of the vertebrae from compression fractures can result in the patient losing height.

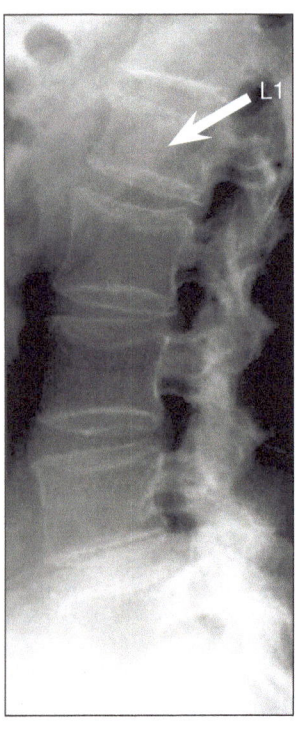 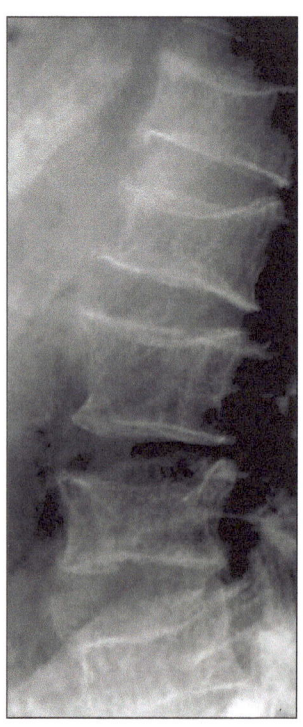

| First fracture | 10 years after first fracture | 20 years after first fracture |

Hip fracture in women without osteoporosis

Figure 2.16. In this study total hip bone mineral density (BMD) and baseline characteristics including physical activity, falls, and strength were assessed in 8065 women aged 65 years or older and these women were then followed-up for up to 5 years after BMD measurement. The graph shows the percentage of women with a hip fracture who did not have osteoporosis at baseline at the total hip, lumbar spine and both sites combined, divided according to age groups. Of the 243 women who developed a hip fracture during follow-up, 54% did not have osteoporosis at the baseline measurement. These findings are consistent with a number of other studies demonstrating that the majority of fragility fractures occur in women who do not have osteoporosis as defined by a T-score ≤-2.5 and emphasize the importance of BMD-independent risk factors as contributors to fracture. Reproduced with permission from Wainwright SA, Marshall LM, Ensrud KE et al. Hip fracture in women without osteoporosis. J Clin Endocrinol Metab 2005; 90:2787–93.

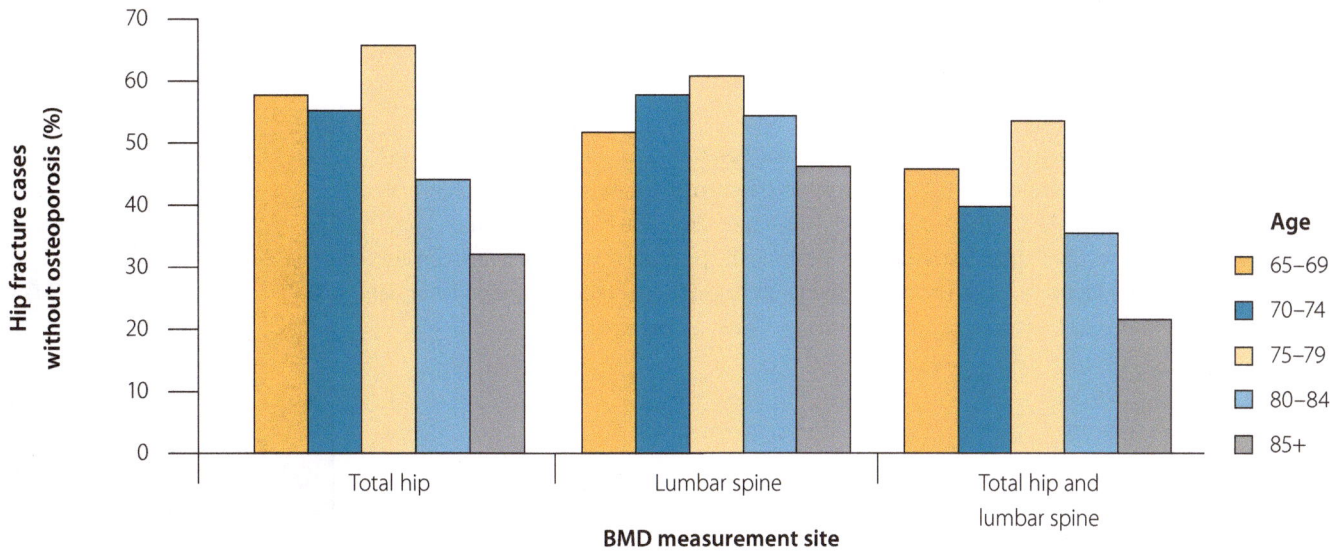

Femoral neck fracture

Figure 2.17. Anteroposterior radiograph showing a fracture of the left femoral neck with some impaction, and mild angulation. The femoral head itself is not dislocated. When examining the radiograph the amount of mal-alignment between the trabecular lines in the femoral head and neck on either side of the fracture line should be examined to determine whether it is a transcervical or subcapital fracture line, with or without displacement. Care should be taken not to miss undisplaced fractures, as a patient may be able to bear weight with some pain and discomfort with the fracture line barely visible on the radiograph. This type of fracture can displace days to weeks after the initial trauma. Courtesy of Professor Pierre Hoffmeyer and Dr Richard Stern, Service d'Orthopédie et de Traumatologie de l'Appareil Moteur, Hôpitaux Universitaires, Geneva, Switzerland.

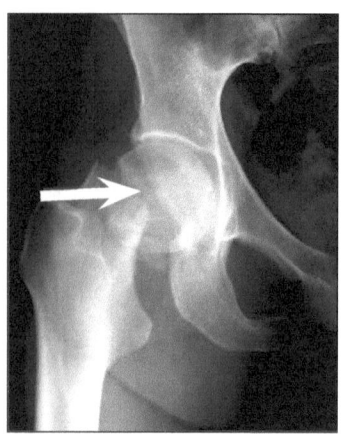

Intertrochanteric fracture of the hip

Figure 2.18. Preoperative anteroposterior radiograph that demonstrates an intertrochanteric left femoral fracture with varus angulation of the distal fracture fragment. Typically, the radiograph reveals a clearly visible crack along the intertrochanteric line, which runs along the base of the femoral neck between the trochanters. Continuous spiral fractures involving the proximal femoral shaft are seen less frequently. Courtesy of Professor Pierre Hoffmeyer and Dr Richard Stern, Service d'Orthopédie et de Traumatologie de l'Appareil Moteur, Hôpitaux Universitaires, Geneva, Switzerland.

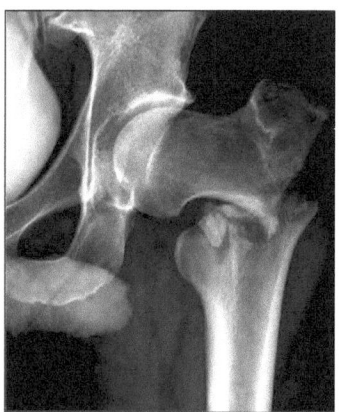

Intertrochanteric and subtrochanteric fracture of the hip

Figure 2.19. Anteroposterior radiograph demonstrating a comminuted fracture in the intertrochanteric/subtrochanteric region of the right hip. A subtrochanteric fracture can be transverse, oblique, or spiral, and occurs at or below the lesser trochanter. Courtesy of Professor Pierre Hoffmeyer and Dr Richard Stern, Service d'Orthopédie et de Traumatologie de l'Appareil Moteur, Hôpitaux Universitaires, Geneva, Switzerland.

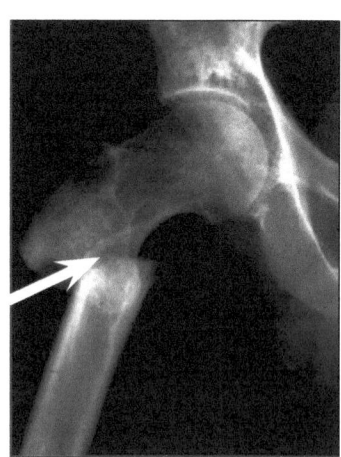

Relationship between hip BMD and hip fracture probability

Figure 2.20. The relationship between osteoporotic fractures, age, and bone mineral density (BMD) at the femoral neck was assessed according to T-scores using dual-X-ray absorptiometry results from published data of a study in Malmö. The results are expressed as a T-score and hip fracture probability in women according to age. For any given T-score the risk is higher with increasing age. The study showed that the risk of hip fracture is increased 14-fold at the age of 50 years in women, but 145-fold at the age of 80 years. From Kanis JA, Johnell O, Oden A et al. Ten year probabilities of osteoporotic fractures according to BMD and diagnostic thresholds. Osteoporos Int 2001; 12:989–95.

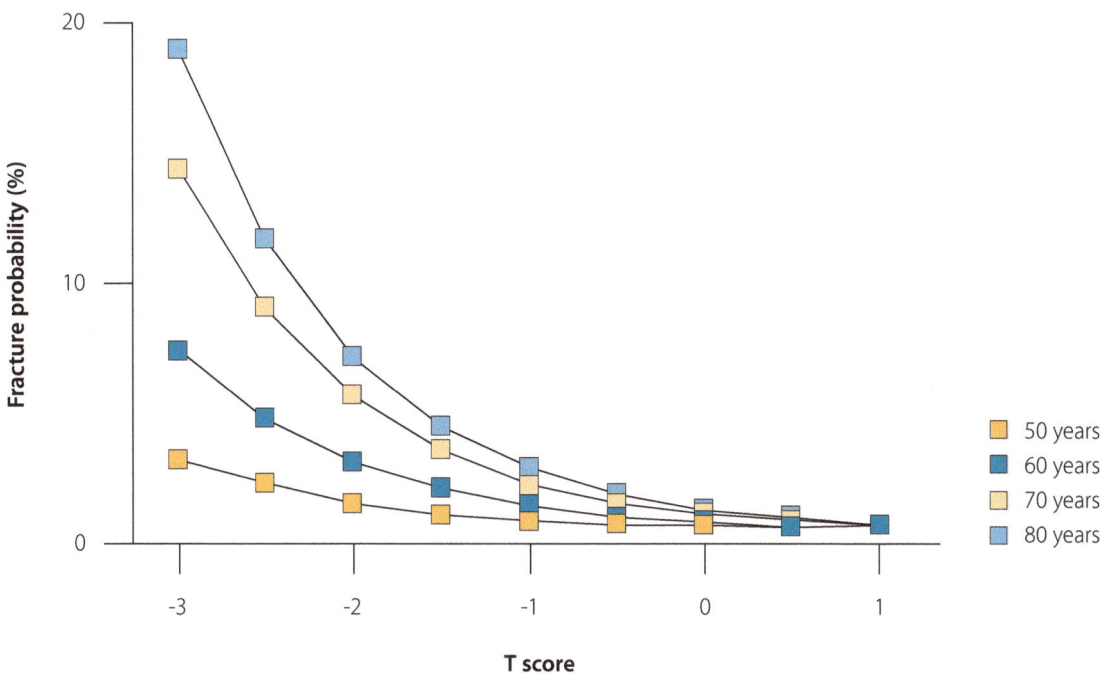

Colles' fracture of the wrist

Figure 2.21. Left wrist radiograph that demonstrates a Colles' fracture of the distal radius. There is also an associated fracture of the ulnar styloid. The classical feature of a Colles' fracture is the 'dinner fork' deformity of the wrist, which is formed of five components: dorsal angulation of the distal fragment, dorsal displacement of the distal fragment, radial deviation of the hand, supination, and proximal impaction. Colles' fractures are typically seen in individuals who have fallen onto an outstretched hand.

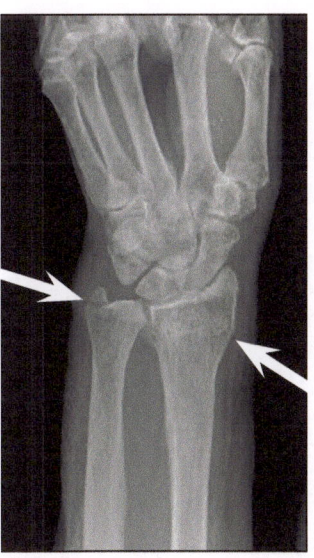

Fracture of the proximal humerus

Figure 2.22. Anteroposterior radiograph demonstrating a proximal humerus fracture (surgical neck) in a 72-year-old woman. Proximal humerus fractures usually result from a fall onto an outstretched hand and are more common in people of middle age or older as the humerus can be weakened by osteoporosis. Four segments of the humerus may be involved: humeral head, lesser or greater tuberosity, surgical neck of the humerus, or anatomical head of the humerus.

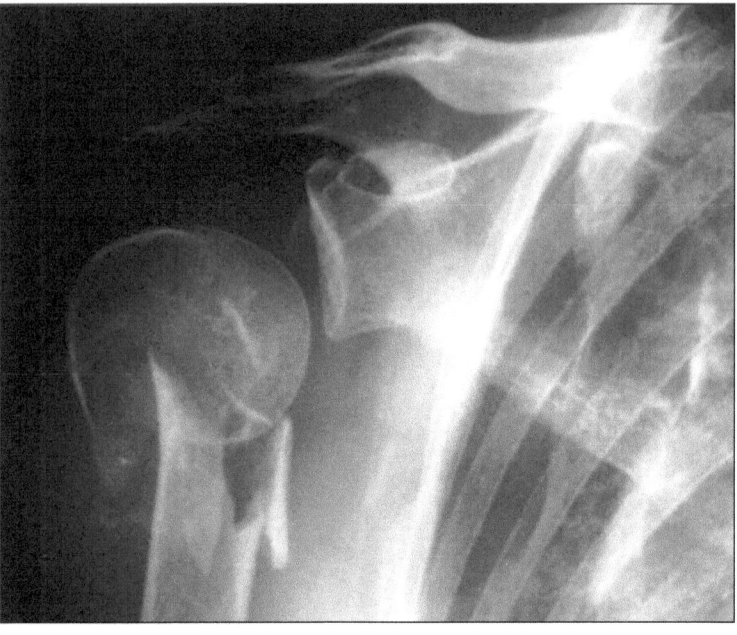

Osteopenia

Figure 2.23. Lateral radiograph of the lumbar spine showing osteopenia. Note the increased radiolucency, and 'picture-framing' of the vertebral bodies owing to loss of trabecular bone and accentuation of the cortical rim. There are also vertical striations of the trabecular bone owing to the relative loss of horizontal trabeculae, and accentuation of the vertical trabeculae. In some cases, the relatively more pronounced decrease in trabecular bone density compared with cortical and subchondral bone densities can give the false impression of increased bone density at the latter sites.

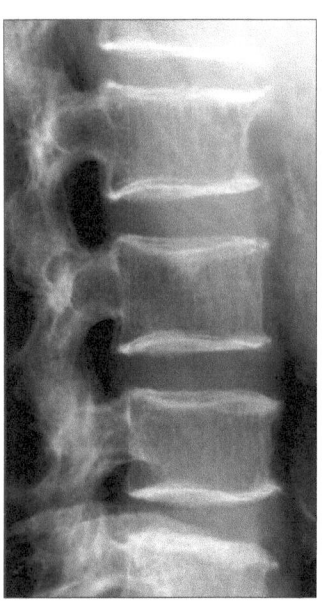

World Heath Organization criteria for the diagnosis of osteoporosis

Figure 2.24. On behalf of the World Health Organization, a group of experts have established definitions and diagnostic criteria for osteopenia and osteoporosis, based on T-scores derived by comparing the patient's bone mineral density (BMD) measurements taken at the spine, hip, or wrist with BMD measurements in healthy white women aged 20–40 years using standard deviations above or below this adult mean. These definitions are invaluable in research to establish the prevalence of osteoporosis, and they are helpful in the screening of patients; however, they should not be used as the sole determinant of treatment decisions. Based on this definition, approximately 30% of postmenopausal women have osteoporosis, with 17% of apparently healthy women in this age group having spinal osteoporosis, 16% having osteoporosis of the femoral neck, and 12% having total hip osteoporosis. Data from World Health Organization. Assessment of fracture risk and its application to screening for postmenopausal osteoporosis. WHO Tech Report Series 1994; 843:1–129.

Diagnosis	T-score
Normal	≥-1.0
Osteopenia	-1 to -2.5
Osteoporosis	≤-2.5
'Established' osteoporosis	≤-2.5 + presence of one or more fractures

Dual-X-ray absorptiometry scan and vertebral body quantitative morphometry

Figure 2.25. (a) Lateral image of the thoracic and lumbar spine obtained by dual-X-ray absorptiometry (DXA), generally visually assessed for vertebral fracture using the Genant SQ grading scheme, **(b)** Electronic digitizing can also be used to calculate different vertebral dimensions. Six-point placement is used in quantitative vertebral morphometry to determine the vertebral dimensions. The dimensions that are derived are the anterior height (*ha*), the central (middle or mid-vertebral) height (*hm*), and the posterior height (*hp*), which can then be used for fracture detection by calculating the wedge ratio (*ha/hp*), the biconcave ratio (*hm/hp*), and the compression ratio (*ha/hp*+1, where 1 indicates the vertebral body above or below).

(a)   **(b)**

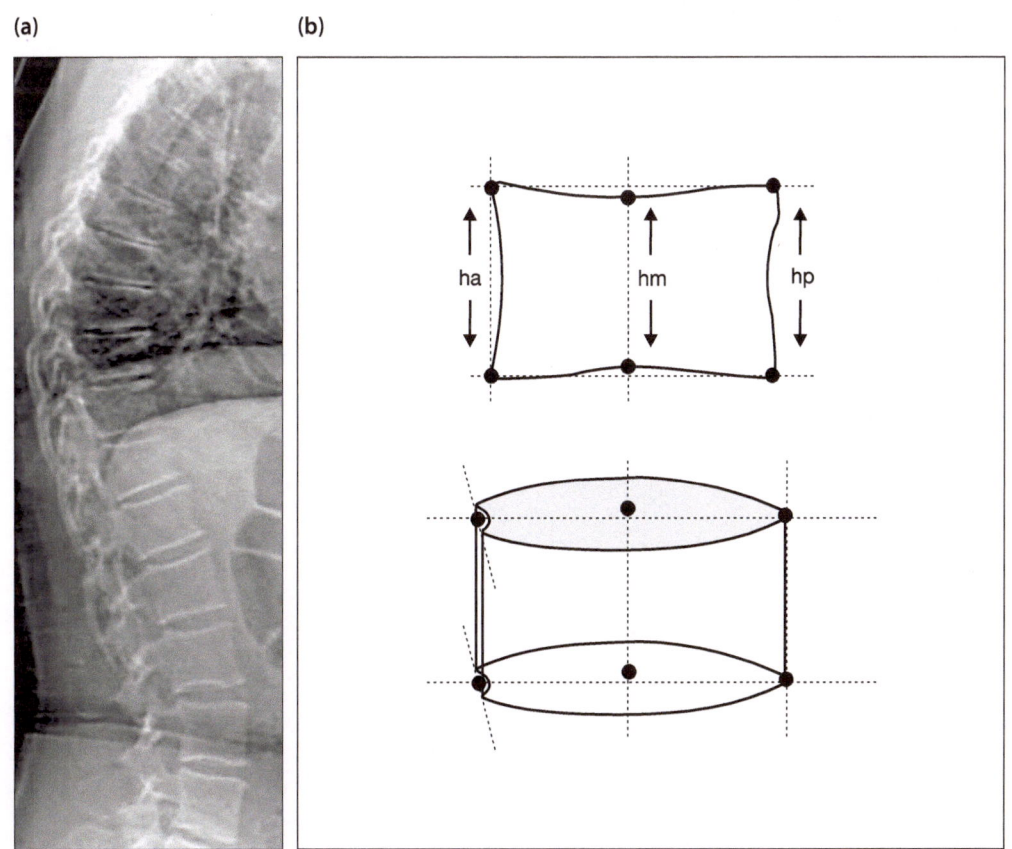

Bone mineral density measurement of the lumbar spine

Figure 2.26. Dual-X-ray absorptiometry image of the lumbar spine of a young healthy adult. Measurements of area, bone mineral content (BMC) and areal bone mineral density (BMD) are generated in L1 to L4 of the lumbar spine and average values are calculated (total). T- and Z-scores are also provided in the print-out. The spine image should be carefully inspected for osteophytes, vertebral fracture, scoliosis or extraskeletal calcification, all of which may artefactually raise the value of BMD.

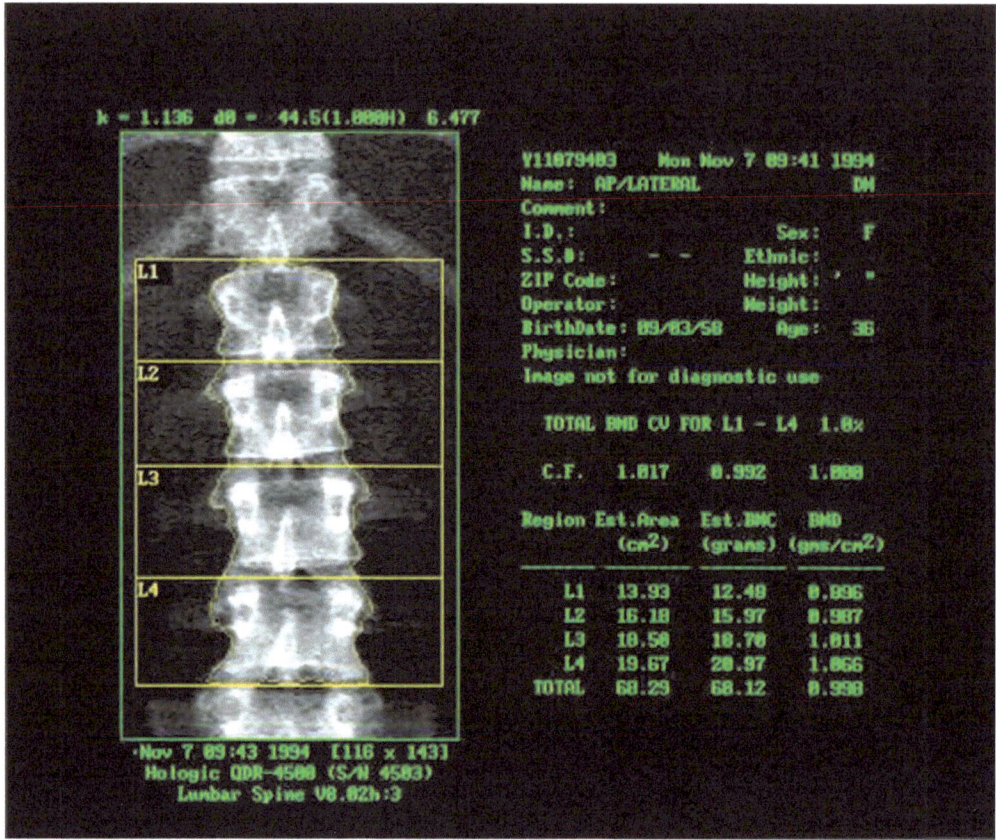

Bone mineral density measurement of the proximal femur

Figure 2.27. Dual-X-ray absorptiometry image of the proximal femur of a young healthy adult. Measurements of bone scanned area, bone mineral content (BMC), and bone mineral density (BMD) are made in the femoral neck **(a)**, trochanter **(b)**, intertrochanteric region **(c)**, and Ward's triangle **(d)** in the proximal femur. T- and Z-scores are also provided in the print-out. The total hip measurement, which is the sum of the femoral neck, trochanter, and intertrochanteric regions, is the preferred site for diagnosis of osteoporosis. Ward's triangle consists predominantly of trabecular bone. Correct positioning of the patient for the scan is important, particularly for follow-up measurements, since differing degrees of rotation can affect the values obtained.

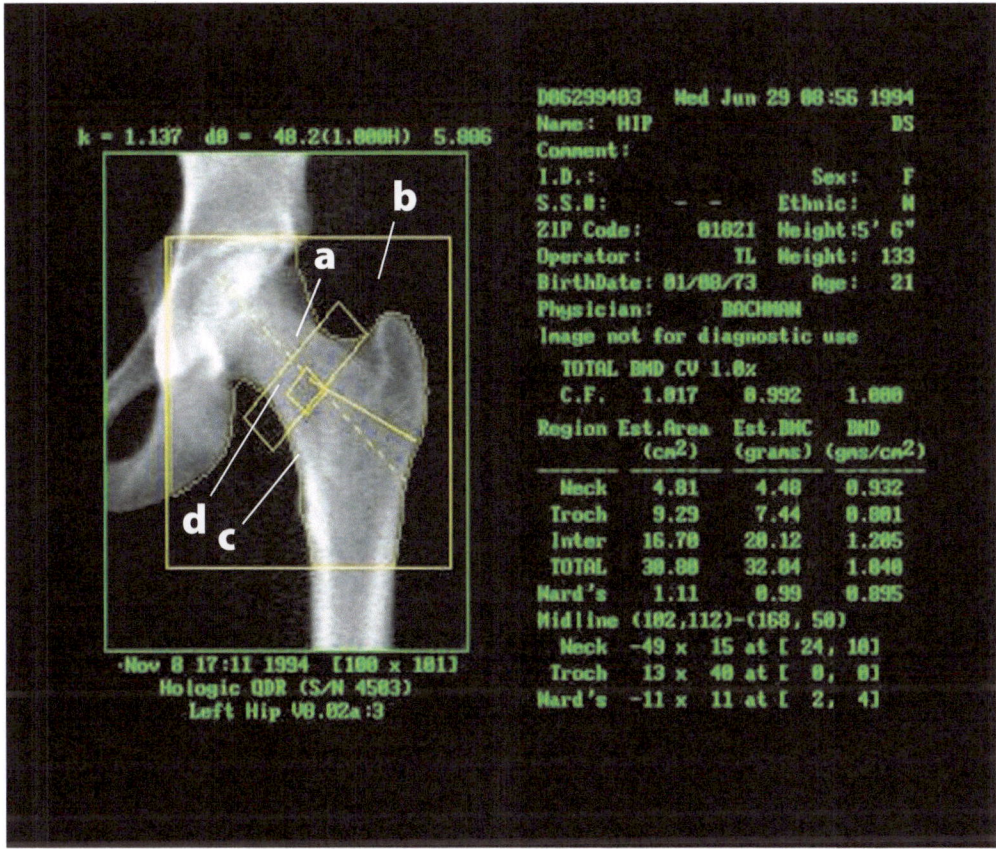

Quantitative ultrasound report

Figure 2.28. Bone density can be measured using quantitative ultrasound, which is different to the more familiar imaging ultrasound techniques used in clinical medicine. The density and quality of the bone is determined by the speed with which sound passes through bone, and the speed of sound (SOS) is reported in m/sec. Bone density and architecture can be determined through attenuation, or the loss of energy from the sound wave as it passes through bone (known as broadband ultrasound attenuation [BUA]), and is reported in db/MHz. When measuring bone density, a coupling medium is required between the sound transducers and skin, and this can be either water (a 'wet' device) or ultrasound gel (a 'dry' device). Most qualitative ultrasound devices measure bone density in the heel, and there are a variety of devices, both wet and dry, available for clinical use. In this figure, the biographical and technical information is found in the center of the report. The numbers after 'Measure' and 'Analysis' refer to the software version used. There is no image produced using this device. The stiffness index is emphasized, although the SOS and BUA are provided in the center section.

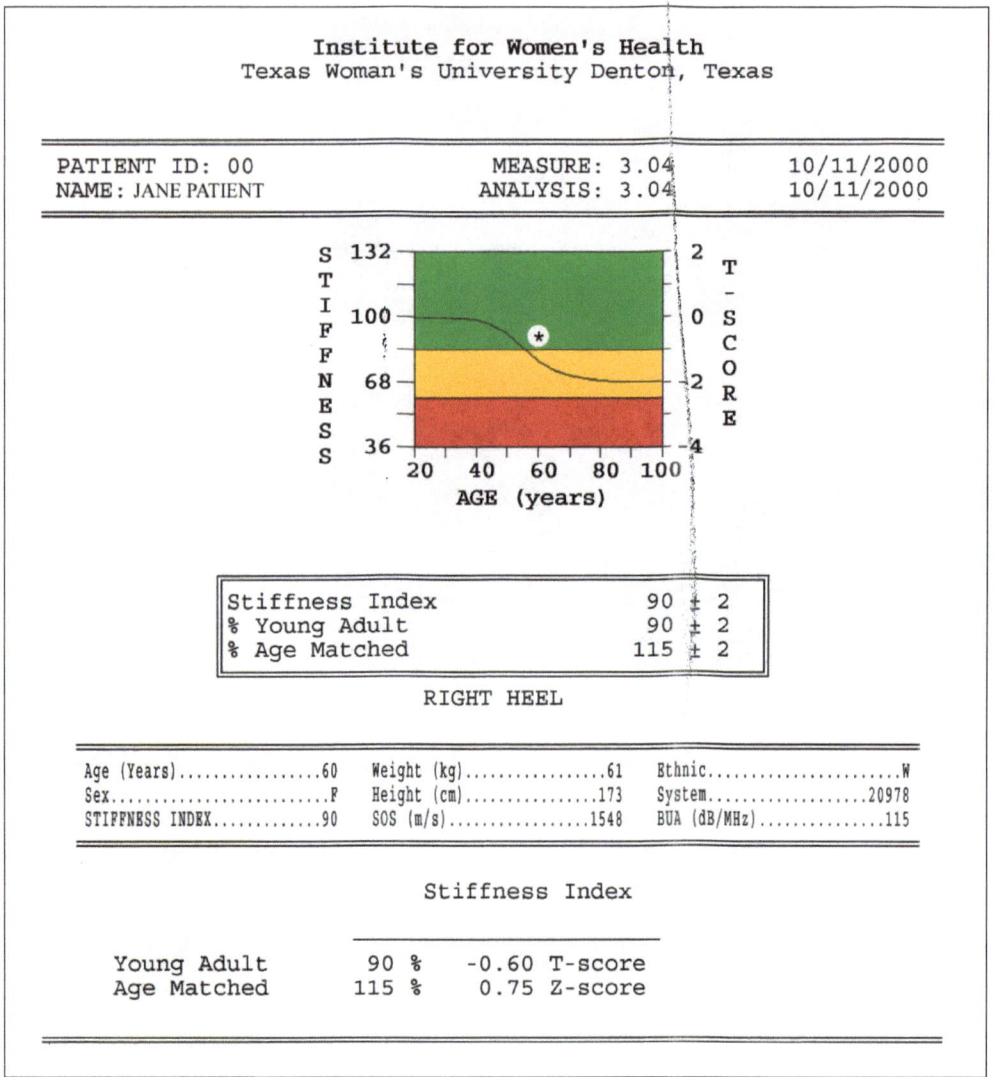

Comparison of various techniques used to measure bone mineral density

Figure 2.29. A comparison of the various techniques used to measure bone mineral density (BMD) is shown. BMD measurements are performed for: diagnostic purposes, to diagnose osteoporosis or osteopenia; for monitoring purposes, to assess changes in BMD over time; and for risk assessment, to predict the risk of fracture. Each of the techniques has advantages and disadvantages. DXA, dual-X-ray absorptiometry.

Technique	Site(s)	Unit of measure	Uses	Particular advantages	Particular disadvantages
Dual-X-ray absorptiometry	Lumbar spine (both lateral and anteroposterior) Proximal femur Total body Forearm Heel Phalanges	Areal density (g/cm^2)	Diagnosis Monitoring	Safe (very low radiation exposure) Precise (reproducibility errors of approximately 0.6–1.5%) and able to detect small changes over time Quick to perform	Anteroposterior spine measurements influenced by degenerative changes and other artefacts Combines trabecular and cortical measurements Two dimensional
Quantitative computed tomography scanning	Lumbar spine Hip Forearm	Volumetric density (g/cm^3)	Diagnosis Monitoring	More sensitive than DXA Slower than DXA Can directly measure trabecular bone loss in the central spine Three dimensional: a true volumetric measurement	Higher radiation exposure than DXA Less precise than DXA More expensive than DXA
Quantitative ultrasound	Heel Patella Tibia	Speed of sound, broadband ultrasound attenuation	Risk assessment	Relatively inexpensive Equipment is easily transportable No radiation exposure	Effectiveness at predicting the risk of fracture is unclear Ability to diagnose osteoporosis is unclear

Genant's semiquantitative grading scale for assessing vertebral fractures

Figure 2.30. Genant et al. have developed a semiquantitative grading scale for assessing vertebral fractures [Genant et al. 1993; Genant & Jergas, 2003]. In this system, the severity of a fracture is assessed solely by visual determination of the extent of vertebral height reduction and morphologic change, and vertebral deformities are differentiated from other, nonfracture, deformities. The approximate degree of height reduction determines the assignment of grades to a vertebra. The type of deformity is not linked to the grading of a fracture. Thoracic and lumbar vertebrae from T4 to L4 are graded as: normal (grade 0); mildly deformed (grade 1: an approximate 20–25% reduction in anterior, middle, and/or posterior height, and a 10–20% reduction in the projected vertebral area); moderately deformed (grade 2: an approximate 25–40% reduction in anterior, middle, and/or posterior height, and 20–40% reduction in the projected vertebral area); and severely deformed (grade 3: an approximately 40% or more reduction in anterior, middle, and/or posterior height, and the projected vertebral area). Grade 0.5 is also sometimes used to designate 'borderline' vertebrae that show some deformation, but which cannot clearly be assigned to grade 1 fractures. Careful attention should also be paid to alterations in the shape and configuration of the vertebrae relative to adjacent vertebrae and expected normal appearances, which can add a strong qualitative, sometimes subjective, aspect to the interpretation. A spinal deformity index can be calculated from these results by adding together all of the grades assigned to the vertebrae. From Genant HK, Jergas M. Assessment of prevalent and incident vertebral fractures in osteoporosis research. Osteoporos Int 2003; 14(Suppl 3):S43–S55.

Grade 0 Normal unfractured vertebrae

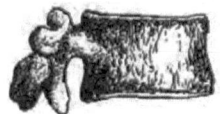

Grade 0.5 Uncertain or questionable fracture with borderline of 20% reduction in anterior middle posterior, or crushed. in all three heights relative to the same or adjacent vertebrae

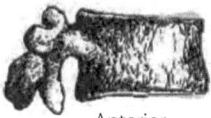 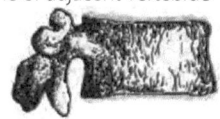

| Anterior | Middle | Crushed |

Grade 1 Mild fracture with 20–25% reduction in anterior middle posterior, or all three heights relative to the same or adjacent vertebrae

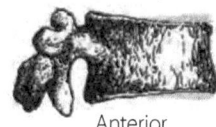 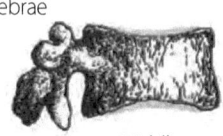 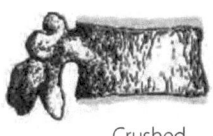

| Anterior | Middle | Crushed |

Grade 2 Moderate fracture with 25–40% reduction in anterior middle posterior, or crushed in all three heights relative to the same or adjacent vertebrae

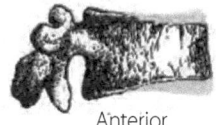 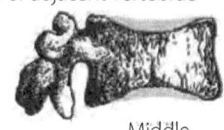 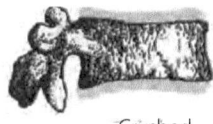

| Anterior | Middle | Crushed |

Grade 3 Severe fracture with >40% reduction in anterior middle posterior, or crushed in all three heights relative to the same or adjacent vertebrae

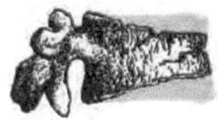 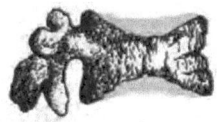 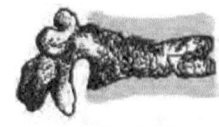

| Anterior | Middle | Crushed |

Coronal magnetic resonance spin echo images of the thoracic vertebrae

Figure 2.31. Coronal magnetic resonance spin echo T1 image (on left) and fast spin echo (FSE) T2 image (on right) demonstrating bilateral diffusely decreased T1 and increased T2-signal intensity within the sacral ala (arrows), which is consistent with bilateral sacral insufficiency fractures. Courtesy of Mikayel Grigoryan, Department of Radiology, University of California, San Francisco, USA.

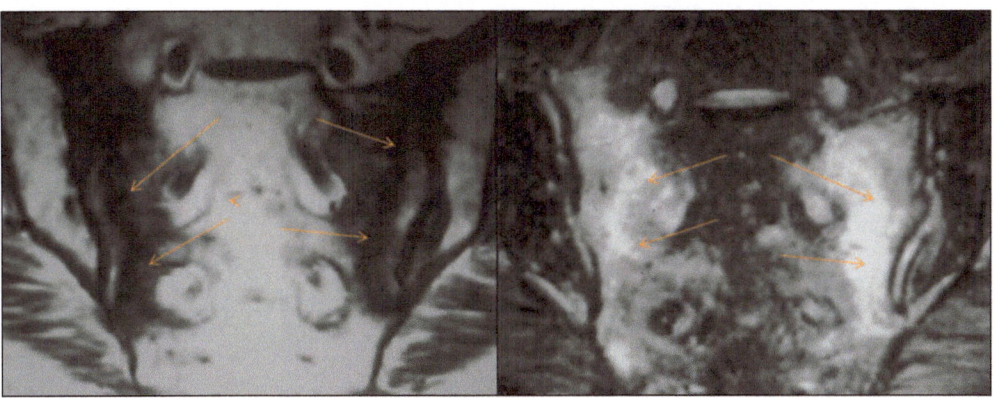

Estimated annual expenditure on fracture management in a UK primary care organization of 100,000 patients

Figure 2.32. In the UK, an estimated 310,000 osteoporotic fractures occur at a cost of GB£1.7 billion. The table shows the estimated costs for a primary care organization (PCO) of 100,000 patients. *Of the 200 patients with radiographic evidence of vertebral fracture, 40 come to clinical attention and are costed. Reproduced with permission from National Osteoporosis Society. Primary Care Strategy for Osteoporosis and Falls. London: National Osteoporosis Society; 2002.

Type of fracture	Predicted number of fractures per PCO of 100,00 patients	Hospital costs (GB£) per fracture	Per PCO (GB£)	Total costs (GB£) per fracture	Total costs per PCO (GB£)
Hip	120	5300	636,000	21,500	2,580,000
Wrist	120	500	60,000	500	60,000
Vertebral*	40 (200)	500	20,000	500	20,000
Other	100	1400	140,000	1400	140,600
Total cost			856,000		2,800,600

Complications and sequelae of osteoporotic fractures

Figure 2.33. There are a number of severe debilitating sequelae of osteoporotic fractures that can lead to permanent disability as listed in this figure. The sequelae can decrease the patient's quality of life considerably, and can even result in death. There are, however, many improved methods of prevention and treatment available.

Hip fractures	Secondary complications of fractures	Adverse effects of vertebral fractures
Permanent disability in more than 30% of patients More than 50% are unable to return to full independence 12–20% die within 1 year after the fracture	Pain Deformity Disability Physical deconditioning caused by inactivity Changes in self-image	Loss of height Kyphosis Crowding of viscera, leading especially to respiratory problems Back pain Prolonged disability Increased mortality

Mortality rates for fracture patients and general population by sex and age group

Figure 2.34. A five-year prospective cohort study was conducted to determine the mortality rates associated with all fracture types in women in a general population, and in female fracture patients by age. The data were collected from a small rural city (Dubbo) in Australia between 1989 and 1992. A total of 356 women had low trauma fractures out of 2413 women. The mortality rate was significantly increased in the fracture patients; for the general female population of all ages, the mortality rate was 37.2 per 1000 person-years compared with 73.0 per 1000 person-years in the fracture patients. The fracture population was significantly older than the general population, and age-adjusted mortality ratios were 1.6 for incident vertebral fractures and 1.8 for prevalent vertebral fractures. These results indicate that there is an association between all major fracture types and increased mortality. Reproduced with permission from Center JR, Nguy TV, Schneider D et al. Mortality after all major types of osteoporotic fracture in men and women: an observational study. Lancet 1999; 353:878–82.

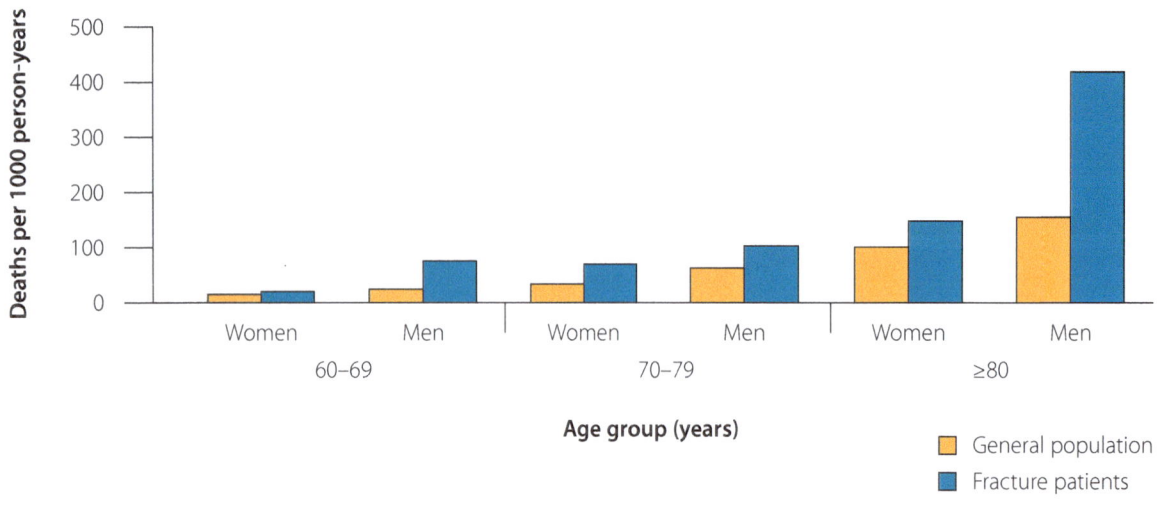

Cumulative survival probability by sex and type of fracture

Figure 2.35. In the same study as Figure 2.34, the cumulative survival probabilities were estimated for the general population, and for the fracture patients by fracture site. Survival was significantly shorter for women in the fracture group than the general population ($p<0.0001$). Other non-hip and vertebral fractures were also associated with significantly shorter survival in women ($p=0.003$). The average life expectancy for this population aged 60 years or older was estimated to be 24 years. In the fracture patients the expected remaining life years for those who had fractures at a younger age were decreased more than for those who had fractures later in life. Therefore, preventive strategies should not only focus on older patients. Reproduced with permission from Center JR, Nguyen TV, Schneider D et al. Mortality after all major types of osteoporotic fracture in men and women: an observational study. Lancet 1999; 353:878–82.

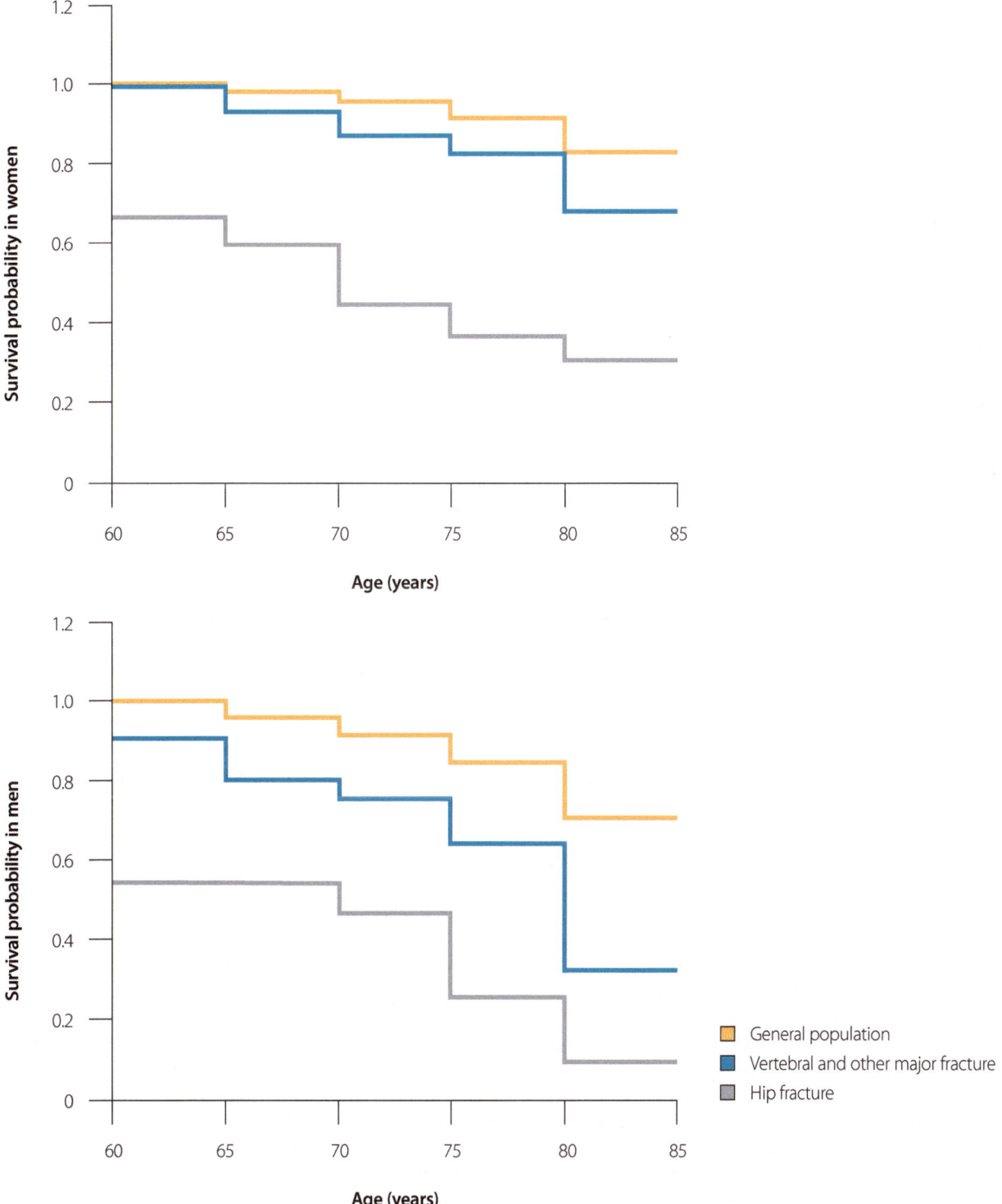

References

Center JR, Nguyen TV, Schneider D et al. Mortality after all major types of osteoporotic fracture in men and women: an observational study. Lancet 1999; 353:878–82.

Compston J. Skeletal effects of drugs. In: Primer on the Metabolic Bone Diseases and Disorders of Mineral Metabolism. 7th edition, Edited by CJ Rosen. Durham NC: American Society for Bome Mineral and Research, 2008; 293-7.

Cooper C. The crippling consequences of fractures and their impact on quality of life. Am J Med 1997; 103:12S–17S.

Cooper C, Atkinson EJ, Jacobsen SJ et al. Population-based study of survival after osteoporotic fractures. Am J Epidemiol 1993; 137:1000–5.

Cooper C, Melton LJ 3rd. Epidemiology of osteoporosis. Trends Endocrinol Metab 1992; 3:224–9.

Cui LH, Choi JS, Shin MH et al. Prevalence of osteoporosis and reference data for lumbar spine and hip bone mineral density in a Korean population J Bone Mineral Metab, 2008; 26:609–17.

Cummings SR, Melton LJ 3rd. Epidemiology and outcomes of osteoporotic fractures. Lancet 2002; 359:1761–7.

Cummings SR, Nevitt MC, Browner WS et al. Risk factors for hip fracture in white women. N Engl J Med 1995; 332:767–73.

Dargent-Molina P, Douchin MN, Corer C et al. Use of clinical risk factors in elderly women with low bone mineral density to identify women at higher risk of hip fracture: the EPIDOS prospective study. Osteoporos Int 2002; 13:595–9.

De Laet CE, Pols HA. Fractures in the elderly: epidemiology and demography. Baillieres Best Pract Res Clin Endocrinol Metab 2000; 14:171–9.

Dennison E, Cooper C. Epidemiology of osteoporotic fractures. Horm Res 2000; 54(Suppl 1):58–63.

Fujiwara S, Nakamura T, Orimo H et al. Development and application of a Japanese model of the WHO fracture risk assessment tool (FRAX™). Osteoporos Int 2008; 19:429–35.

Garton MJ, Robertson EM, Gilbert FJ et al. Can radiologists detect osteopenia on plain radiographs? Clin Radiol 1994; 49:118–22.

Genant HK, Cann CE, Ettinger B et al. Qualitative computed tomography of vertebral spongiosa: A sensitive method for detecting early bone loss after oophorectomy. Ann Intern Med 1982; 97:699–705.

Genant HK, Engelke K, Fuerst T et al. Noninvasive assessment of bone mineral and structure: state of the art. J Bone Miner Res 1996; 11:707–30.

Genant HK, Jergas M. Assessment of prevalent and incident vertebral fractures in osteoporosis research. Osteoporos Int 2003; 14(Suppl 3):S43–S55.

Genant HK, Siris E, Crans GG et al. Reduction in vertebral fracture risk in teriparatide-treated postmenopausal women as assessed by spinal deformity index. Bone 2005; 37:170–4.

Genant HK, Wu CY, van Kuijk C et al. Vertebral fracture assessment using a semiquantitative technique. J Bone Miner Res 1993; 8:1137–48.

Glüer CC, Hans D. How to use ultrasound for risk assessment: a need for defining strategies. Osteoporos Int 1999; 9:193–5.

Greenspan SL, Myers ER, Maitland LA et al. Fall severity and bone mineral density as risk factors for hip fracture in ambulatory elderly. JAMA 1994; 271:128–33.

Jiang G, Ferrar L, Barrington N et al. Standardised quantitative morphometry: a modified approach for quantitative identification of prevalent vertebral deformities Osteoporosis Int 2007; 18: 1411–9.

Johnell O, Oden A, De Laet C et al. Biochemical indices of bone turnover and the assessment of fracture probability. Osteoporos Int 2002; 13:523–6.

Kanis JA et al. on behalf of the World Health Organization Scientific Group. Assessment of osteoporosis at the primary health care level. Technical Report. World Health Organization Collaborating Centre, University of Sheffield, UK. 2008.

Kanis A, Johnell O, Oden A et al. FRAX™ and the assessment of fracture probability in men and women from the UK. Osteoporos Int 2008a; 19:385–397.

Kanis J, Johnell O. Requirements for DXA for the management of osteoporosis in Europe. Osteoporos Int 2005; 16:229–38.

Kanis J, Johansson H, Johnell O et al. Alcohol intake as a risk factor for fracture. Osteoporos Int 2005a; 16:737–2.

Kanis J, Johnell O, Oden A. Smoking and fracture risk: a metaanalysis. Osteoporos Int 2005b; 16:155–62.

Kanis JA, Borgstrom F, De Laet C et al. Assessment of fracture risk. Osteoporos Int 2005c; 16:581–9.

Kanis JA, Johnell O, Oden A et al. Ten year probabilities of osteoporotic fractures according to BMD and diagnostic thresholds. Osteoporos Int 2001; 12:989–95.

Kanis JA, Johnell O, Oden A et al. Long-term risk of osteoporotic fracture in Malmö. Osteoporos Int 2000; 11:669–74.

Klotzbuecher CM, Ross PD, Landsman PB et al. Patients with prior fractures have an increased risk of future fractures: a summary of the literature and statistical synthesis. J Bone Miner Res 2000; 15:721–39.

Lau EM. Epidemiology of osteoporosis. Best Pract Res Clin Rheumatol 2001; 15:335–44.

Lindsay R, Silverman SL, Cooper C et al. Risk of new vertebral fracture in the year following a fracture. JAMA 2001; 285:320–3.

Marottoli RA, Berkman LF, Cooney LM Jr. Decline in physical function following hip fracture. J Am Geriatr Soc 1992; 40:861–6.

Marshall D, Johnell O, Wedel H. Meta-analysis of how well measures of bone mineral density predict occurrence of osteoporotic fractures. BMJ 1996; 312:1254–9.

Melton LJ 3rd. How many women have osteoporosis now? J Bone Miner Res 1995; 10:175–7.

National Osteoporosis Foundation. 1996 and 2015 Osteoporosis Prevalence Figures: State-by-State Report. Washington, DC: National Osteoporosis Foundation; 1997.

National Osteoporosis Society. Position Statement on the Reporting of Dual Energy X-ray Absorptiometry (DXA) Bone Mineral Density Scans. London: National Osteoporosis Society; 2002a.

National Osteoporosis Society. Primary Care Strategy for Osteoporosis and Falls. London: National Osteoporosis Society; 2002.

Nevitt MC, Cummings SR. Type of fall and risk of hip and wrist fractures: the Study of Osteoporotic Fractures. J Am Geriatr Soc 1993; 41:1226–34.

O'Neill TW, Felsenberg D, Varlow J et al. The prevalence of vertebral deformity in European men and women: the European Vertebral Osteoporosis Study. J Bone Miner Res 1996; 11:1010–8.

Papaioannou A, Watts NB, Kendler DL et al. Diagnosis and management of vertebral fractures in elderly adults. Am J Med 2002; 113:220–8.

Ray NF, Chan JK, Thamer M et al. Medical expenditures for the treatment of osteoporotic fractures in the United States in 1995: report from the National Osteoporosis Foundation. J Bone Miner Res 1997; 12:24–35.

Ross PD. Clinical consequences of vertebral fractures. Am J Med 1997; 103(Suppl 2A):30S–42S.

Schlaich C, Minnie HW, Bruckner T et al. Reduced pulmonary function in patients with spinal osteoporotic fractures. Osteoporos Int 1998; 8:261–7.

Siris ES, Miller PD, Barrett-Connor E et al. Identification and fracture outcomes of undiagnosed low bone mineral density in postmenopausal women: results from the National Osteoporosis Risk Assessment. JAMA 2001; 286:2815–22.

Torgerson DJ, Campbell MK, Thomas RE et al. Prediction of perimenopausal fractures by bone mineral density and other risks factors. J Bone Miner Res 1996; 11:293–7.

Wainwright SA, Marshall LM, Ensrud KE et al. Hip fracture in women without osteoporosis. J Clin Endocrinol Metab 2005; 90:2787–93.

Wei TS, Hu CH, Wang SH et al. Fall characteristics, functional mobility and bone mineral density as risk factors of hip fracture in the community-dwelling ambulatory elderly. Osteoporos Int 2001; 12:1050–5.

World Health Organization. Assessment of fracture risk and its application to screening for postmenopausal osteoporosis. WHO Tech Report Series 1994; 843:1–129.

Chapter 3
Bone quality and strength

Patrick Ammann and René Rizzoli

Bone strength is the maximal load that can be applied before a fracture occurs. It is influenced by a number of different factors, such as mass, geometry, architecture, and intrinsic bone tissue quality (Figure 3.1). Bone tissue quality is related to microstructure, to the degree of mineralization, and to matrix characteristics, such as the orientation and chemical structure of the collagen fibers. The aim of antiosteoporotic treatments is to improve bone strength, and thus decrease the risk of fracture (Figure 3.2). In humans, the end point used to evaluate bone strength is fracture occurence; large numbers of patients are required to demonstrate significant reductions as a result of therapeutic intervention. Fracture is not only caused by decreased bone mineral mass, or alteration of the microarchitecture, but is also related to falls, which can occur as a result of loss of balance, inappropriate protective responses, or muscle weakness (Figure 3.3). Thus, careful and specific investigation in animal models to examine the effects of antiosteoporotic treatments on bone strength (Figure 3.4) and its determinants is of major importance.

Determinants of bone strength
Areal bone mineral density
Currently, the most commonly used noninvasive measurement for the diagnosis of osteoporosis is measurement of areal bone mineral density (BMD) by dual-X-ray absorptiometry (DXA). BMD is a major determinant of bone strength and BMD values obtained at the proximal femur and lumbar spine are used to diagnose osteoporosis by applying criteria established by the World Health Organization (WHO) [World Health Organization Study Group, 1994]. Most of the clinical studies on inhibitors of bone resorption, such as bisphosphonates, selective estrogen receptor modulators (SERMs), or estrogen, have shown some association between an increase of areal BMD and a decreased risk of fracture (Figures 3.5–3.6), but the relationship between these is very inconsistent [Hauselmann & Rizzoli, 2003]. Thus, raloxifene and alendronate treatment are both associated with a reduction of vertebral fracture, but the effect on BMD is less pronounced with raloxifene treatment (+3%) than with alendronate (+8%) [Riggs & Melton, 2002]. Fluoride treatment has been shown to induce major increments of BMD (+10%/year), but does not consistently reduce the incidence of vertebral fracture. This may be explained, at least partially, by the modification of bone mineral when, fluoride is incorporated into hydroxyapatite, leading to increased brittleness of the bone. In untreated bone, *ex vivo* studies performed on human samples have indicated an excellent correlation between BMD and bone strength, as evaluated by shear test of the femoral neck [Bouxsein et al. 1999], or compression of the vertebrae (Figure 3.5) [Granhed et al. 1989]. These *ex vivo* studies indicate that BMD predicts approximately 66–74% of the variance of bone stregth. BMD is not a volumetric (mass per volume) density, but an areal density (mass per area) (Figure 3.7). Indeed, BMD corresponds to the ratio of bone mineral content (hydroxyapatite) and bone scanned area. Thus, this variable integrates not only the amount of mineral, but also the dimensions of bone. The high level of prediction of bone strength by areal BMD could be explained, at least partially, by the fact that bone size is integrated in this measurement.

Bone geometry
Among the determinants of bone strength, bone geometry, such as external diameter and cortical thickness, plays a major role. Mechanical studies have demonstrated that increasing the external diameter of a cylinder greatly increases its resistance to flexion (Figures 3.8–3.9). An increase in cortical thickness also improves bone strength, but to a lesser extent. The outer diameter of the long bones predicts up to 55% of the variance of the bone strength [Bonjour et al.1999; Ammann et al. 1998; Turner, 2002; Turner & Burr, 1993].

Stimulators of bone formation, such as insulin-like growth factor-1 (IGF-1), growth hormone [Andreassen et al. 1995], or parathyroid hormone (PTH), stimulate periosteal apposition [Ejersted et al. 1993], and increase the external diameter of long bones (Figures 3.10–3.11). This expansion of the outer diameter of long bone is associated with a marked increment of bone strength. An increase in cortical thickness may also be observed with antiresorptive therapy, and results from inhibition of endosteal bone resorption.

After ovariectomy, expansion of the external diameter of the long bones and femoral neck is observed, which results in increased bone strength, a compensatory reaction to the decrease in bone mass and to the alteration of trabecular architecture [Bagi et al. 1997]. These changes are associated with increased plasma IGF-1, which may stimulate periosteal apposition, and thus explain the outer diameter expansion. In contrast to ovariectomy, isocaloric low protein intake (50% of the minimal amount necessary to maintain normal metabolism and bone mass) decreases bone strength and BMD [Ammann et al. 2000] (Figures 3.12–3.14). In this situation, the compensatory mechanism of periosteal expansion does not take place [Bourrin et al. 2000]. Furthermore changes in tissue quality may also be implicated [Hengsberger et al. 2005].

Expansion of bone diameter is also observed in humans. During growth, the bone diameter is influenced by nutritional factors and physical exercise. In elderly men, an expansion of bone outer diameter occurs, and with PTH treatment an increased bone area can be detected. An excess of growth hormone, as in acromegaly, also increases bone size. Thus, an increase in bone size is possible in adults, but its specific role as a determinant of the risk of fracture remains to be determined.

Bone microarchitecture

Sex hormone deficiency is associated with alteration of the connectivity of trabecular structures, including decreased trabecular number, increased trabecular separation, modification of trabecular shape from plates to rods, and alteration of connectivity. These aspects of bone microarchitecture can be assessed by histomorphometry or by microcomputed tomography (microCT) (Figure 3.15).

Histomorphometry allows a two-dimensional evaluation of the microarchitecture, thus providing information on bone quality, including structure and turnover, which is independent of bone mass (Figures 3.16–3.18). Using a tetracycline double-labeling procedure dynamic parameters such as bone formation could be evaluated (Figure 3.19). Histomorphometric analysis is usually performed on transiliac bone biopsies. In practice, it is used to exclude the diagnosis of osteomalacia, to identify high and low bone turnover and to assess the effects of treatments on bone quality and safety.

MicroCT allows one to examine the three-dimensional microarchitecture of bone as well as the relative bone volume and trabecular thickness (Figures 3.20–3.21). It does not, however, allow us to analyze unmineralized tissue and bone cells. Increasing vertebral fracture severity (as measured by semi-quantitative analysis) is characterized by deterioration in bone microarchictecture [Delmas et al. 2005]. This deterioration is a continuous and progressive process which helps to explain the accelerated cascade of fracture risk in patients with severe vertebral fracture. Alterations in trabecular structure contribute to changes in bone strength (Figure 3.22). Ovariectomy can reduce bone strength and bone mass; however, significant modifications of vertebral bone strength can be detected before any decrease in BMD. Dissociation between these two variables may be due to early alteration of the microarchitecture (perforation and/or disappearance of trabeculae) without major effects on BMD. Therefore, the mechanical properties of trabecular bone are dominated by volume fraction, and the extent of anisotropy. In fact, most morphologic properties calculated from three-dimensional microCT images, such as trabecular thickness, trabecular spacing, connectivity, and structural index, are to some extent correlated with volume fraction.

Bone tissue quality

One parameter that should be considered is the degree of mineralization (Figure 3.23). Increased bone strength is observed with bisphosphonate therapy, without significant changes in bone mass or trabecular bone volume as evaluated by histomorphometry [Boivin et al. 2000]. A more homogeneous distribution of mineralization is observed, which may contribute to the increase in BMD, and in bone strength [Chavassieux et al. 1997] (Figure 3.24). The reduced rate of bone remodeling may also be implicated [Bourrin et al. 2002].

Clinical studies indicate that markers of bone remodeling are independent predictors of the risk of fracture. By changing the distribution of stress in relation to the volume of bone in a phase of remodeling, a high remodeling rate could decrease mechanical strength (Figure 3.25). Alternatively, decreased bone remodeling may influence trabecular bone geometry, and the degree of mineralization of the matrix formed under treatment. The latter is a function of the time available for mineralization of the newly formed matrix [Boivin & Meunier, 2001].

A nanoindentation technique is used to investigate tissue quality by measuring both hardness, and elasticity, of dry and wet bone tissue with a high spatial resolution. Nanoindentation involves impressing a pyramidal diamond tip into a material, and simultaneously recording force and displacement with milli-Newton and nanometer resolution. From the resulting force–displacement curves, hardness (the maximal force per unit area), and indentation modulus (a purely elastic property) can be calculated (Figure 3.26). The nanoindentation method allows the mechanical properties of single bone structural units to be quantified. There are few results currently available, but local elastic properties of bone structural units were found to vary significantly among individuals and anatomic locations [Rho et al. 1997]. Little correlation was found between age and the elastic properties of bone tissue [Hoffler et al. 2000]. Since bone is constantly remodeled in young and older individuals, there is recently remodeled and old bone in adjacent areas. This could explain a poor correlation between age and heterogeneity in an individual. Nanoindentation has the potential to become a major new tool in the assessment of tissue quality, and elucidation of mechanisms by which osteoporotic treatments improve bone strength. In the future, it could be applied to bone biopsy samples to determine the contribution of tissue quality to bone fragility.

Evaluation of bone strength

Bone strength is evaluated by various methods for different parts of the skeleton: compression of the vertebral body or of the proximal tibia, three- or four-point bending test of the long bones (eg, tibia, femur, or humerus), and shear test of the femoral neck (Figures 3.27–3.28). For the biomechanical tests, a load–deflection curve is recorded, allowing the calculation of various components: stiffness, by measuring the slope of the linear part of the curve; ultimate strength, by measuring the highest load applied before fracture; and energy absorbed (toughness), by measuring the area under the curve (Figure 3.29). Other parameters can be derived, for example, the yield point, which corresponds to the transition from an elastic to a plastic or irreversible deformation of the sample. All these different tests are well described, and their reproducibility (3–5%) is evaluated by measuring the variation between right and left bone samples in the same animal, or the difference between adjacent vertebrae. These measurements can be used to evaluate the severity of bone fragility as well as the integrated effect of treatment on the various determinants of bone strength.

Determinants of bone mechanical properties

Figure 3.1. Bone strength is determined by bone geometry, cortical thickness, porosity, trabecular bone morphology, and intrinsic properties of bone tissue. Bone remodeling results in modification of major determinants of bone strength, such as mass, microarchitecture (trabecular volume, connectivity, and thickness), geometry (outer diameter, and cortical thickness), and factors related to the intrinsic mechanical quality of bone tissue (mineralization, cortical porosity, collagen fibril orientation and links, and microdamage). Selective alterations of all these determinants during bone remodeling characterize bone mechanical properties. Careful assessment of all the determinants of bone strength (bone tissue included) should be considered in the pathophysiology of osteoporosis, and in the mechanisms of action of antiosteoporotic drugs.

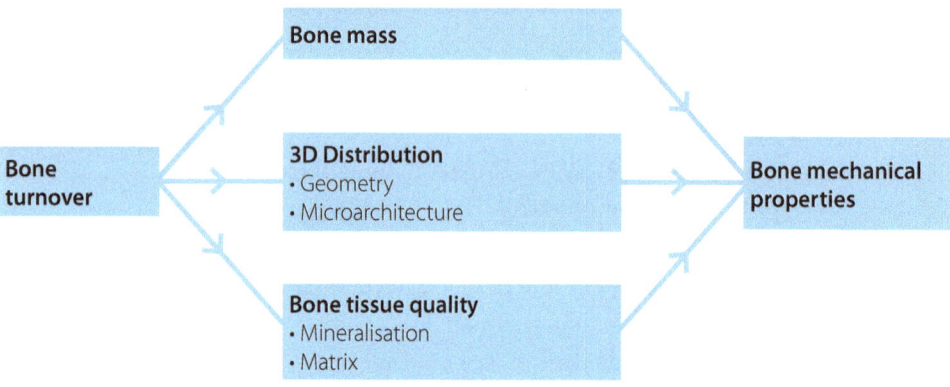

Vertebral fracture between two osteoporotic vertebrae

Figure 3.2. Osteoporosis is defined as a decrease in bone mass, and alteration of microarchitecture leading to increased bone fragility. The major complication of the disease is an increased risk of fracture occurring with low-energy trauma. The presence of a fracture is not, however, required for the diagnosis of osteoporosis.

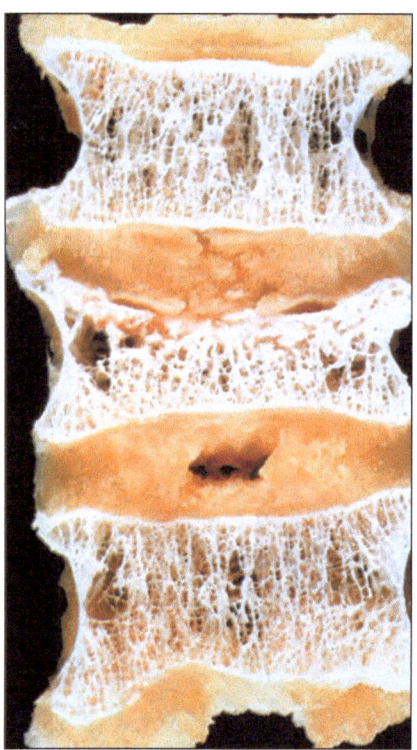

Determinants of fracture risk

Figure 3.3. Osteoporotic fracture results from decreased bone mineral mass, changes in microarchitecture, or geometry (which are influenced by hormones, nutrition, exercise, and lifestyle factors), and low-energy trauma as a result of loss of balance, inappropriate protective responses, or muscle weakness. Bone strength is discussed in Figure 3.1.

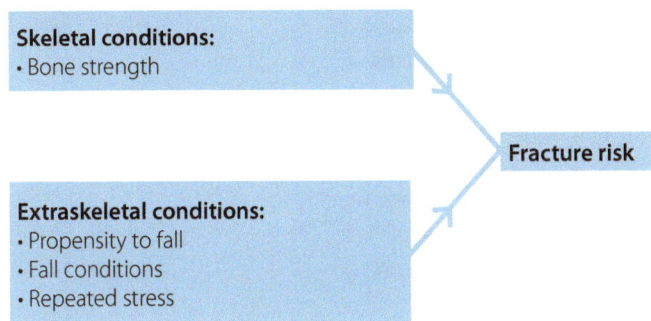

Effects of anticatabolic and anabolic agents on determinants of bone strength

Figure 3.4. Bone strength, a determinant of resistance to fracture, depends on bone mineral density, geometry, microarchitecture, bone turnover rate and properties of the bone at the material level. Despite comparable antifracture efficacy, anticatabolics and bone anabolic agents are likely to modify the various determinants of bone strength in very different ways. Parathyroid hormone (PTH) influences microarchitecture while bisphosphonates alter material-level bone properties, with probable opposite effects on remodeling space. Raloxifene primarily improves the material stiffness at the cortical level. Strontium ranelate improves bone strentgh by positively influencing all the different determinants. Adapted from Brennan TC, Rizzoli R, Ammann P. Selective modification of bone quality by PTH, pamidronate or raloxifene. J Bone Miner Res 2009; 24:800–8, and Bain SD, Jerome C, Shen I et al. Strontium ranelate improves bone strength in ovariectomized rat by positively influencing bone resistance determinants. Osteoporosis Int 2009; 20:1417–28.

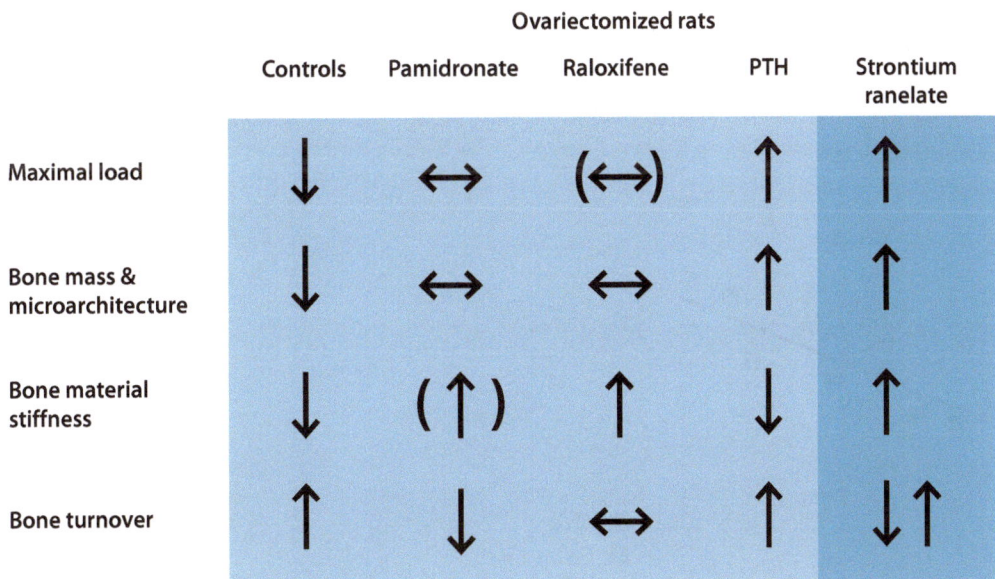

Relationship between bone strength and BMD in clinical and preclinical studies

Figure 3.5. Currently, the major noninvasive measurement available for the diagnosis of osteoporosis is measurement of areal bone mineral density (BMD) by dual-X-ray absorptiometry (DXA). BMD is considered a predictor of bone strength. *Ex vivo* studies performed on human and animal specimens have indicated an excellent correlation between bone strength as evaluated by shear test of the femoral neck and BMD of the proximal femur. **(a)** In a human study of 26 people, a correlation coefficient of 0.92 was found between the ultimate force at fracture and femoral trochanter BMD. The *ex vivo* studies on human material indicate that bone mineral content predicts approximately 66–74% of the variance in bone strength. Data from Bouxsein ML, Coan BS, Lee SC. Prediction of the strength of the elderly proximal femur by bone mineral density and quantitative ultrasound measurements of the heel and tibia. Bone 1999; 25:49–54. **(b)** In preclinical studies (pigs, monkeys, rats, mice), BMD predicts 50–75% of the variance of the ultimate strength. Bone strength was assessed using compression of vertebral body and BMD measured by DXA. In ovariectomized (OVX) osteoporotic rats treated with a stimulator of bone formation (insulin like growth factor-1 [IGF-1]), an inhibitor of bone resorption (bisphosphonate pamidronate [APD]), or a combination of both treatments, for all the groups 62% of the variance of the ultimate strength was predicted by BMD. Data from Ammann P, Rizzoli R, Meyer JM et al. Bone density and shape as determinants of bone strength in IGF-1 and/or pamidronate-treated ovariectomized rats. Osteoporos Int 1996; 6:219–27.

(a) Human

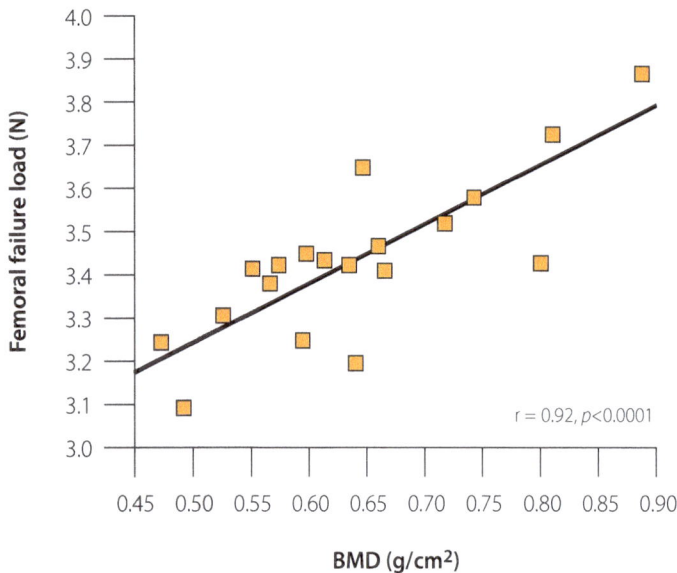

(b) Rats model
Lumbar spine

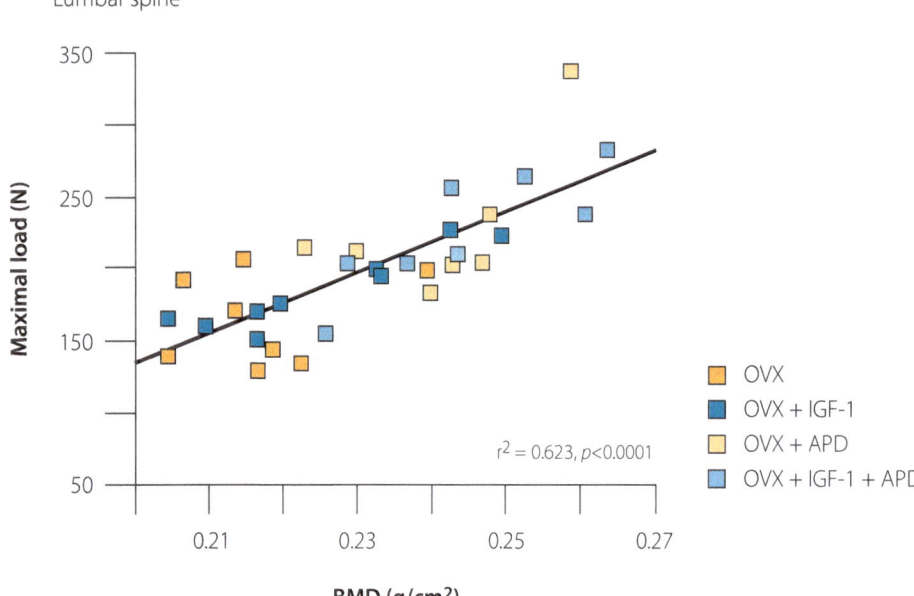

Prediction of hip fracture risk

Figure 3.6. Assessment of bone mineral density (BMD) and the bone resorption rate can be combined to predict hip fracture risk in the elderly. Elderly women (n = 126; mean age 82.5 years) who sustained a hip fracture during a mean 22-month follow-up were age-matched with three controls who did not fracture. Low BMD was defined according to the World Health Organization definition [World Health Organization Study Group, 1994] as a value lower than −2.5 standard deviation (SD) of the young adult mean. High bone resorption was defined by carboxy-terminal cross-linked telopeptides of type 1 collagen (CTX), or free deoxypyridinoline (D-Pyr) values higher than the upper limit (mean+2 SD) of the premenopausal range. Women with both low hip BMD and high bone resorption rate were at a higher risk of hip fracture than women with either low hip BMD or high bone resorption alone. Increased bone resorption was found to predict hip fracture independently of bone mass. Reproduced with permission from Garnero P, Hausherr E, Chapuy MC et al. Markers of bone resorption predict hip fracture in elderly women: the EPIDOS Prospective Study. J Bone Miner Res 1996; 11:1531–8.

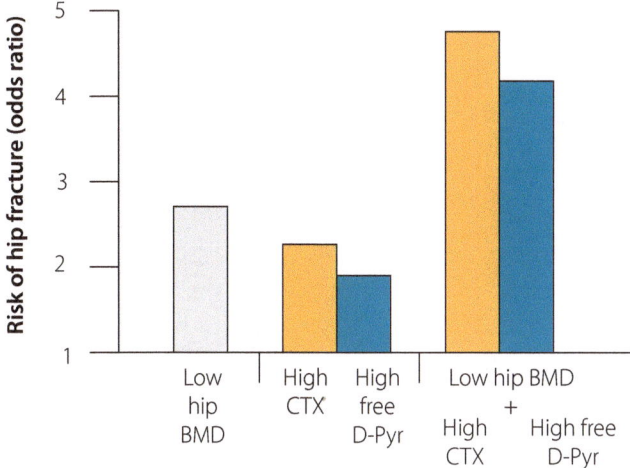

Areal BMD measurement integrates information concerning bone mass and dimensions

Figure 3.7. Bone mineral density, (BMD) is an areal density and not a volumetric density. This leads to the indirect introduction of the anteroposterior dimension of the bone investigated. The fact that BMD reflects bone density and dimension could explain why BMD is a predictor of bone strength. This is represented in the figure; material added with identical volumetric density on the anterior posterior direction increase BMD values but not when added on the lateral sides. BMC, bone mineral content.

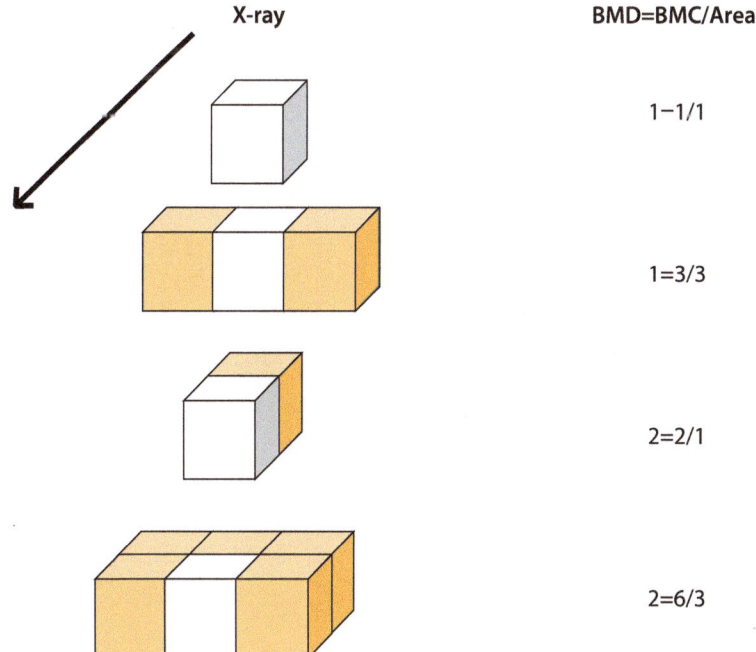

The importance of bone dimensions

Figure 3.8. Among the determinants of bone strength, the dimension of the bones play a major role. For example, it is easier to crush a rectangular cardboard box than to crush a cardboard tube of identical mass. For the same amount of material, bending resistance is higher for a cardboard tube than for a cardoard box. In a similar way, the cylindrical shape of bones helps to provide maximum strength for a given volume.

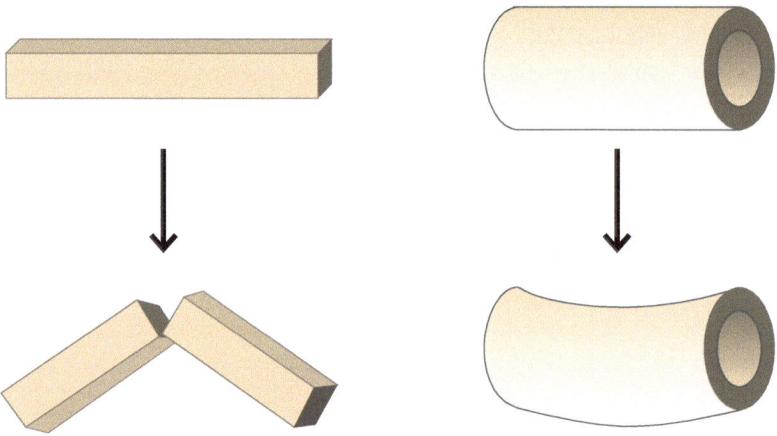

Size, microarchitecture and bone stength

Figure 3.9. The external diameter of bone and cortical thickness are key components of bone dimensions. From mechanical evidence, it is demonstrated that increasing the external diameter of a cylinder strongly increases the resistance to flexion. The enlargement of the cortical thickness also improves bone strength, but to a lesser extent. The filling of the cylinder with the same material (ie, increased cortical thickness) results in an increment of bending resistance lower than one with the same mass located away from the center of the cylinder (ie, increased external diameter). The combination of increments of outer diameter and cortical thickness results in an additive effect on bone strength. Adapted from Turner CH. Toward a cure for osteoporosis: reversal of excessive bone fragility. Osteoporos Int 1991; 2:12–9.

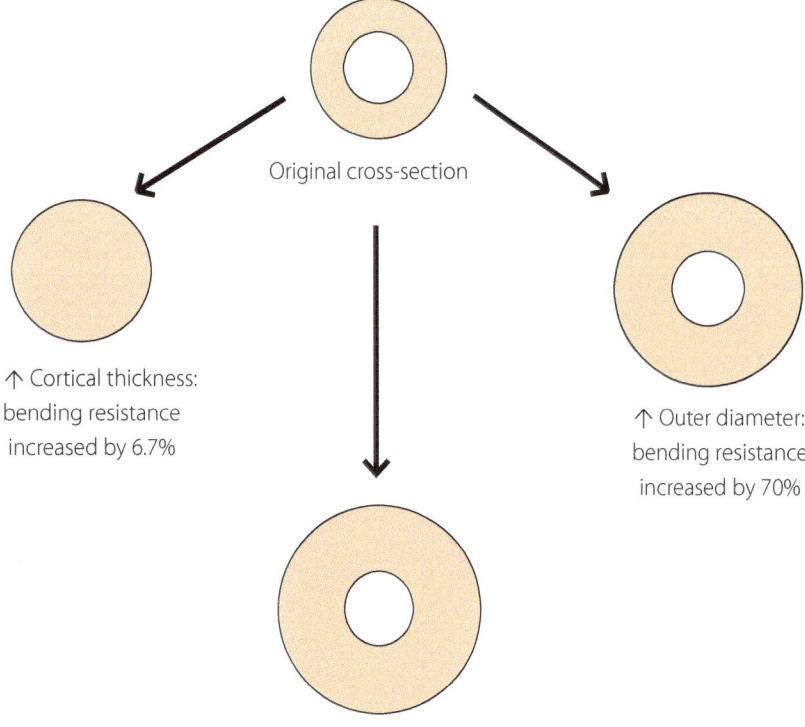

Original cross-section

↑ Cortical thickness:
bending resistance
increased by 6.7%

↑ Outer diameter:
bending resistance
increased by 70%

↑ Cortical thickness and outer diameter:
bending resistance increased by 255%

The effect of insulin-like growth factor-1 on the external diameter of long bones

Figure 3.10. Treatment with insulin-like growth factor-1 (IGF-1), an anabolic agent, stimulates periosteal apposition, and increases the external diameter of the long bones. This expansion of the outer diameter of long bones is associated with an increase of bone strength. An increase in cortical thickness may also be observed with antiresorptive therapy (bisphosphonate pamidronate [APD]), and results from inhibition of endosteal bone resorption, thereby contributing to the improvement in bone strength. These results are from ovariectomized (OVX) six-month-old rats treated for six weeks with APD and/or IGF-1. The midshaft tibia dimensions (diameters, cortical thicknesses and bone surfaces) were measured using image analysis after section performed at the level of the middle of the tibia. The results are expressed as means ± SEM (mm or mm^2). *p <0.05 compared with OVX. Reproduced with permission from Ammann P, Rizzoli R, Bonjour JP. Preclinical evaluation of new therapeutic agents for osteoporosis. In: Osteoporosis: Diagnosis and Management. Edited by PJ Meunier. London: Martin Dunitz, 1998; 257–73.

	OVX (vehicle)	OVX + APD	OVX + IGF-1	OVX + APD+IGF-1
External diameter	2.81 ± 0.04	2.82 ± 0.05	2.91 ± 0.03	2.98 ± 0.06*
Cortical thickness	0.63 ± 0.01	0.68 ± 0.02*	0.64 ± 0.02	0.71 ± 0.01*
Bone surfaces	4.51 ± 0.12	4.55 ± 0.16	4.61 ± 0.11	5.10 ± 0.13*

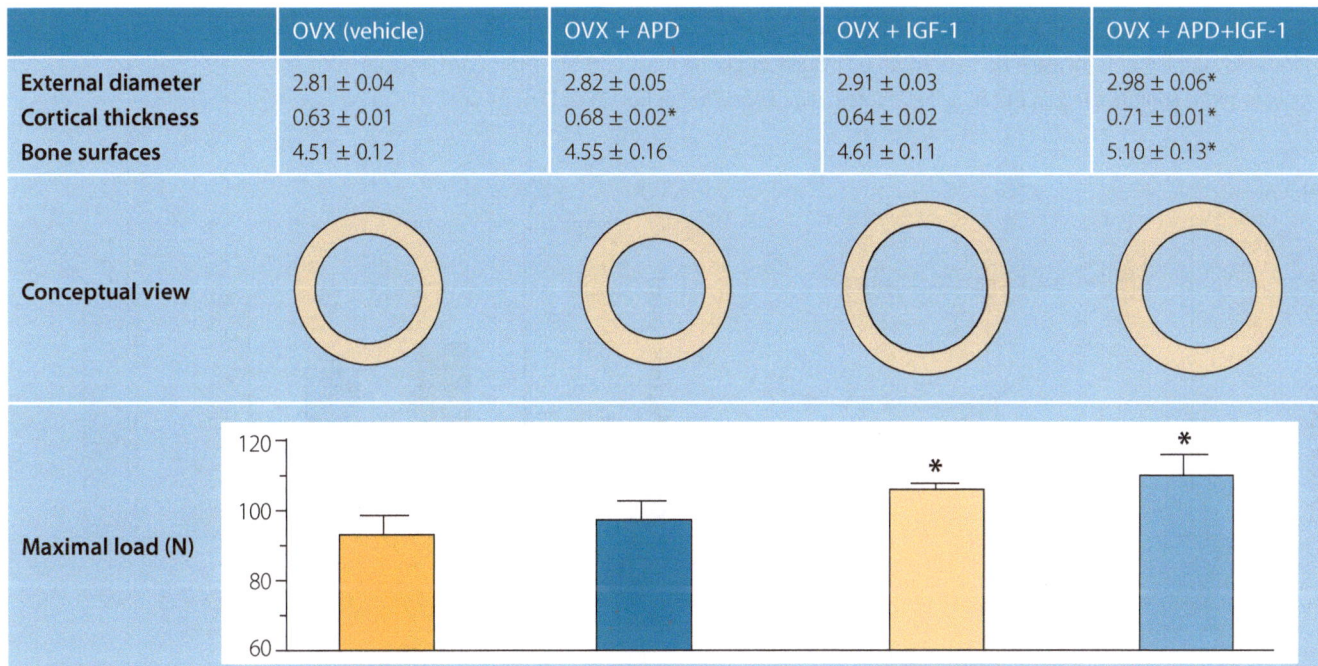

Relative modification of geometry and maximal load

Figure 3.11. Treatment with insulin-like growth factor-1 (IGF-1), an anabolic agent, or with strontium ranelate stimulates periosteal apposition and increases the external diameter of the long bones. Such an increment of external diameter was not observed with antiresorptive therapy (bisphosphonate pamidronate [APD]). Under IGF-1 and strontium ranelate treatment an increase of outer diameter by 4% resulted in a threefold increase of bone strength. In preclinical studies with pamidronate no significant increment of external diameter and bone strength were observed. This observation underlines the importance of outer diameter to predict bone strength; a minor increment of outer diameter resulted in a major effect on bone strength. NS, not significant; OVX, ovariectomized rats. Data from Ammann P, Rizzoli R, Meyer JM et al. Bone density and shape as determinants of bone strength in IGF-I and/or pamidronate-treated ovariectomized rats. Osteoporos Int 1996; 6:219–27 and Ammann P, Shen V, Robin B et al. Strontium ranelate improves bone resistance by increasing bone mass and improving architecture in intact female rats. Bone Miner Res 2004; 19:2012–20.

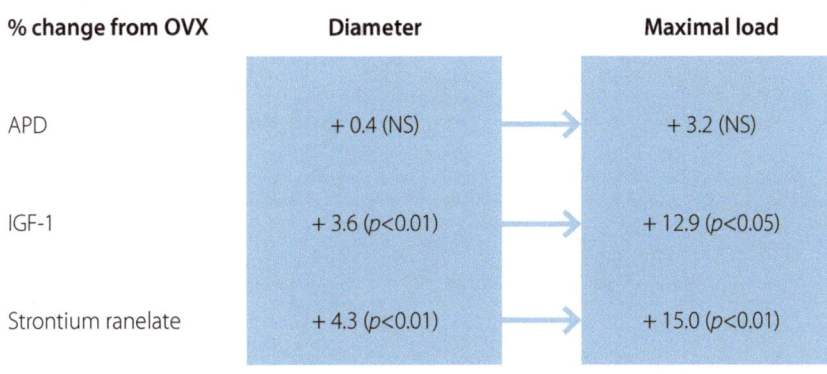

% change from OVX	Diameter	Maximal load
APD	+ 0.4 (NS)	+ 3.2 (NS)
IGF-1	+ 3.6 (p<0.01)	+ 12.9 (p<0.05)
Strontium ranelate	+ 4.3 (p<0.01)	+ 15.0 (p<0.01)

Effect of essential amino acids on vertebrae in ovariectomized rats fed on a low-protein diet

Figure 3.12. The effect of administration of an isocaloric essential amino acid supplement (EAA; at a dose of 5%) on **(a)** bone mineral density (BMD), **(b)** cortical bone thickness and **(c)** bone strength was studied in adult female rats made osteoporotic by ovariectomy (OVX), and fed a low-protein diet. In (a), OVX rats fed a low-protein diet were treated with EAA; the study also included control rats (SHAM) fed a 15% casein diet, and treatment was started at week 10 (dotted line). In (b) and (c), measurements were performed at 10 weeks (basal) and 16 weeks of EAA supplementation. Cortical bone thickness was measured by microtomographic histomorphometry at the level of the L4 vertebra, and ultimate strength at the level of the vertebral body by an axial compression test. The administration of an EAA supplement in OVX osteoporotic rats, fed a low-protein diet, restored bone strength. This was associated with prevention of further bone loss, and with increased cortical thickness resulting from reduced resorption of trabeculae at the endocortical surface. *$p < 0.01$ compared with OVX rats fed a low-protein diet; †$p < 0.01$ compared with basal and OVX rats fed a low-protein diet. Reproduced with permission from Ammann P, Laib A, Bonjour JP et al. Dietary essential amino acid supplements increase bone strength by influencing bone mass and bone microarchitecture in ovariectomized adult rats fed an isocaloric low-protein diet. J Bone Miner Res 2002; 17:1264–72.

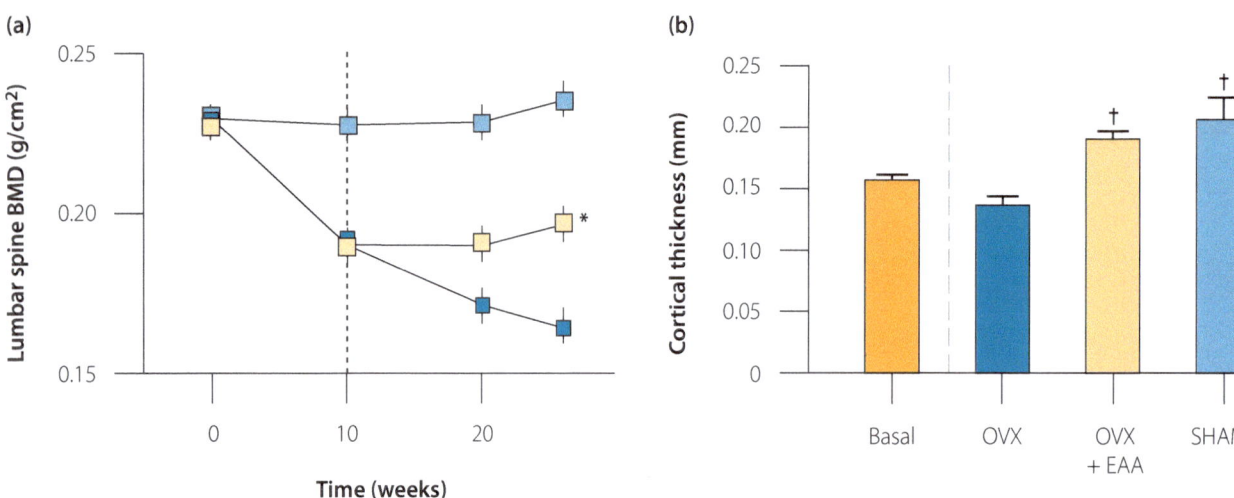

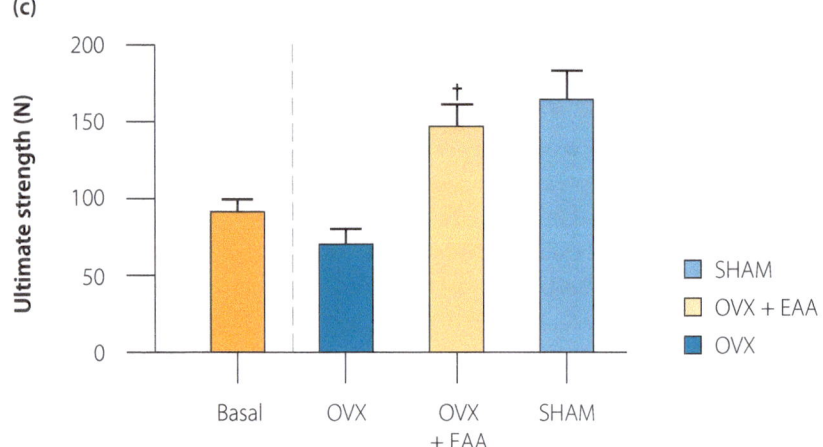

Effect of protein malnutrition and amino acids supplements on bone microarchitecture

Figure 3.13. Low protein diet is associated with decreased trabecular volume, perforation and thinning of trabeculae. The administration of an essential amino acid supplement in osteoporotic rats, fed a low-protein diet, restores bone strength through improvement of the microarchitecture of the vertebra, modifications of bone mineral density and cortical thickness. These modifications were observed in association with an increase in insulin-like growth factor-1 (IGF-1). An IGF-1-mediated process may therefore be involved [Ammann et al. 2002].

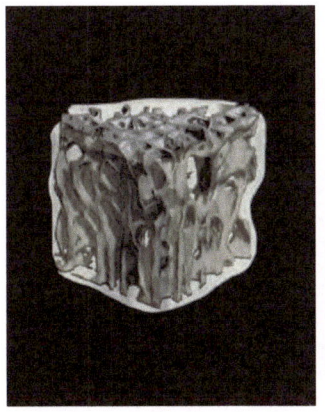 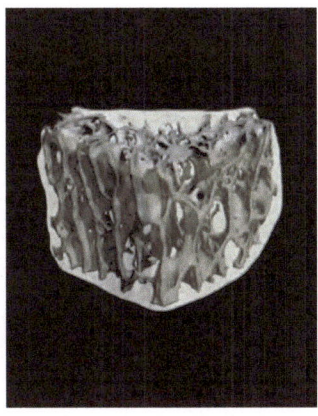 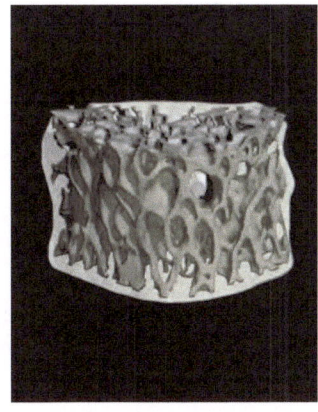

<table>
<tr><td>**Control**</td><td>**Low protein diet**</td><td>**Low protein diet**
Essential amino acid
supplements</td></tr>
</table>

Effect of protein malnutrition and amino acid supplements on bone tissue quality:
a nanoindentation study

Figure 3.14. Ovariectomy and a low protein diet have a deleterious effect on bone tissue quality as evaluated at the level of the vertebral body. In one study, rats were randomly allocated to one of two groups receiving 2.5% casein (OVX 2.5) or 2.5% casein and 5.0% essential amino acids (OVX 2.5 + EAA 5.0). The administration of an EAA supplement in ovariectomized osteoporotic rats, fed a low-protein diet, corrected the decreased working energy. This benefit may help to restore mechanical properties of bone. $*p < 0.05$. Adapted from Hengsberger S, Ammann P, Legros B et al. Intrinsic bone tissue properties in adult rat vertebrae: modulation by dietary protein. Bone 2005; 36:134–41.

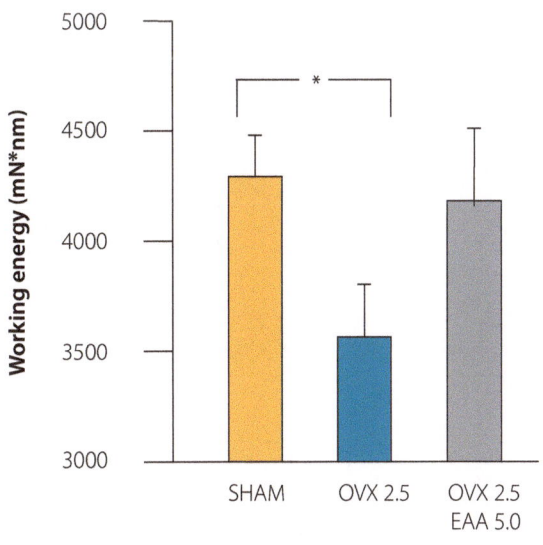

Effects of pamidronate or PTH on microarchitecture and bone strength in ovariectomized rats

Figure 3.15. Effects of curative treatments with pamidronate or parathyroid hormone (PTH) on microarchitecture and bone strength in ovariectomized (OVX) rats. Bone strength, a determinant of resistance to fracture, depends on mass, geometry and microarchitecture. Anticatabolic agents prevent further deterioration of bone mass and microarchitecture. Bone anabolic agents increase bone mass and improve microarchitecture. Bone strength is expressed as the mean ± SEM. Adapted from Brennan TC, Rizzoli R, Ammann P. Selective modification of bone quality by PTH, pamidronate, or raloxifene. J Bone Miner Res 2009; 24: 800–8.

Control

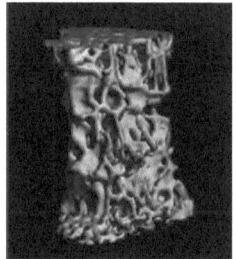

Mean bone strength
= 303.5 ± 27.3 N

OVX

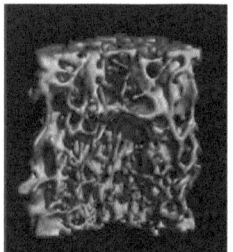

Mean bone strength
= 215.8 ± 11.3 N

OVX + bisphosphonate pamidronate

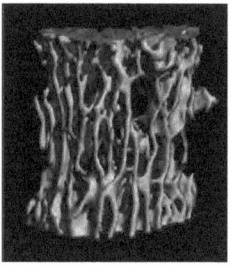

Mean bone strength
= 321.1 ± 18.1 N

OVX + PTH

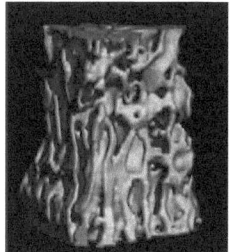

Mean bone strength
= 404.9 ± 25.0 N

Key measurements in bone histomorphometry

Figure 3.16. In 1987 a committee from the American Society of Bone and Mineral Reseach proposed a standardized nomenclature of histomorphometric parameters. The abbreviations and parameters in the table below are expressed in three dimension and represent those commonly reported from histomorphometric analyses. *Calculated from the trabecular bone area and volume and the length of the bone marrow interface; †Calculated from the mean apposition rate and the mineralizing surfaces. BMD, bone mineral density. Adapted from Parfitt AM, Drezner MK, Glorieux FH et al. Bone histomorphometry: standardization of nomenclature, symbols and units. J Bone Miner Res 1987; 2:595–610.

Parameters of bone structure	Abbreviation (unit)	Description
Parameters expressing the amount of bone		
Cancellous bone volume	Cn-BV/TV (%)	The percentage of spongy bone tissue including mineralized bone and osteoid
Total bone volume	BV/Tt.CV (%)	This is an estimate of bone mass
Cortical width	Ct.Wi (mm)	The thickness of the cortices
Wall thickness	W.Th (mm)	The width of complete trabecular bone
Parameters reflecting trabecular bone microarchitecture		
Trabecular thickness*	Tb.Th (mm)	The width of the trabeculae
Trabecular separation*	Tb.Sp (mm)	The distance between trabeculae
Trabecular number*	Tb.N (mm)	The density of trabeculae
Parameters of bone formation		
Static parameters		
Osteoid volume	OV/BV (%)	The fraction of trabecular tissue which is not calcified
Osteoid surface	OS/BS (%)	The percentage of total trabecular surface covered with osteoid
Osteoid thickness	O.Th (μm)	The average width of osteoid seams
Dynamic parameters		
Mineral apposition rate	MAR (μm/day)	It expresses the rate of progression of the mineralization front
Mineralizing surfaces	dLS/BS (%) sLS/BS (%) LS/BS (%)	The extent of double, single or total tetracycline labeled surfaces expressed as a percentage of total trabecular bone surfaces
Derived parameters		
Bone formation rate†	Cn-BFR/BS ($μm^3/μm^2$/day)	The amount of mineralized bone made per unit of trabecular bone per day
Adjusted apposition rate	Aj.AR (μm/day)	The amount of mineralized bone made per day per unit of osteoid-covered surface
Formation period	FP (days)	The mean time needed to build a new bone structural unit
Mineralization lag time	Mlt (days)	The mean interval between the deposition of osteoid and the mineralization
Activation frequency	Cn-BFR/W.Th (per year)	Number of bone-multicellular units born per year. Represents the probability that a new cycle of bone remodeling will start on the bone surface
Bone resorption parameters		
Eroded surface	ES/BS (%)	The percentage of trabecular bone surface eroded
Osteoclast number	N.Oc/BS	Number per millimeter of trabecular surface
Erosion depth	E.De (μm)	Derived from the number of eroded lamellae in each resorption cavity and the lamellar thickness

Effect of strontium ranelate on the histology of the proximal tibia

Figure 3.17. The effect of strontium ranelate on the proximal tibia of intact rats **(a)** compared with controls **(b)** is shown. With strontium ranelate treatment the trabecular bone volume (BV/TV) increased by 41.5%, the trabecular thickness increased by 12.2%, the trabecular number increased by 28.5%, and trabecular spacing was reduced by 27.5% compared with the control.

(a)   **(b)**

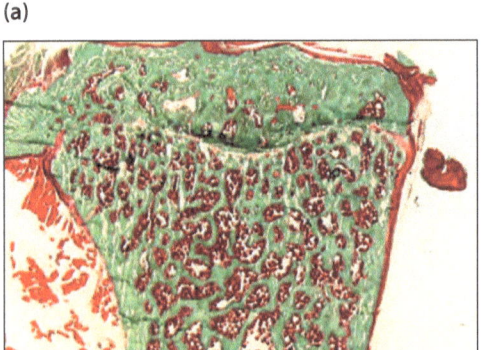 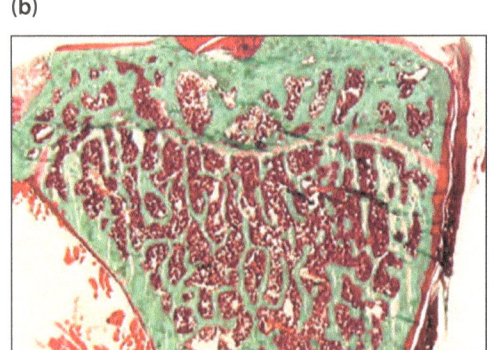

Microcracks in bone

Figure 3.18. The presence of microcracks could theoretically contribute to deterioration of intrinsic tissue quality. This was studied in 36 female dogs divided into three groups: control group treated with saline vehicle for 12 months, risedronate-treated group, and alendronate-treated group. The doses of risedronate and alendronate were six times those used in humans. **(a)** A microcrack with a sharp border in the right femoral neck cortex from a risedronate-treated dog, and **(b)** focal microdamage area showing cracks without sharp borders in the third lumbar vertebral body from an alendronate-treated dog. One year of treatment with risedronate or alendronate significantly suppressed trabecular remodeling in vertebrae and ilium without impairment of mineralization, and significantly increased microdamage accumulation in all skeletal sites measured. However, bone strength was not affected. Stained *en bloc* with basic fuchsin. Original magnification ×98. Reproduced with permission from Mashiba T, Turner CH, Hirano T et al. Effects of suppressed bone turnover by bisphosphonates on microdamage accumulation and biomechanical properties in clinically relevant skeletal sites in beagles. Bone 2001; 28:524–31.

(a)   **(b)**

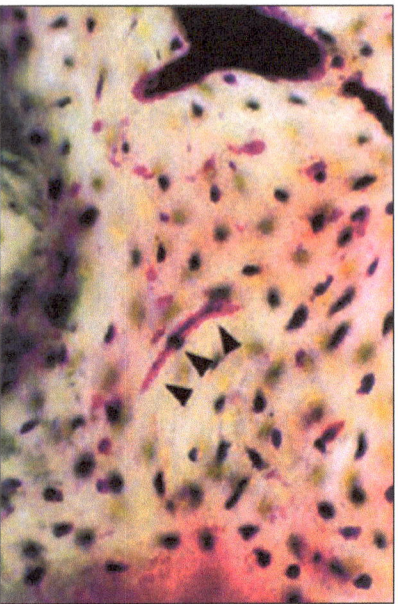 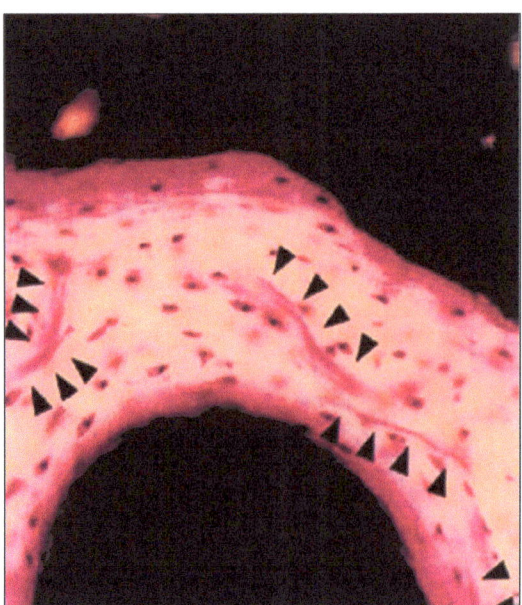

Dynamic bone histomorphometric analysis

Figure 3.19. Dynamic bone histomorphometric analysis allows us to evaluate, beside the microarchitecture, the mineralizing surfaces, mineral apposition rate and the bone formation rate. **(a)** Bone resorption by osteoclast and bone formation by osteoblast. **(b)** The space between two tetracycline labeling allows to quantify mineralization rate and bone formation.

(a)　　　　　　　　　**(b)**

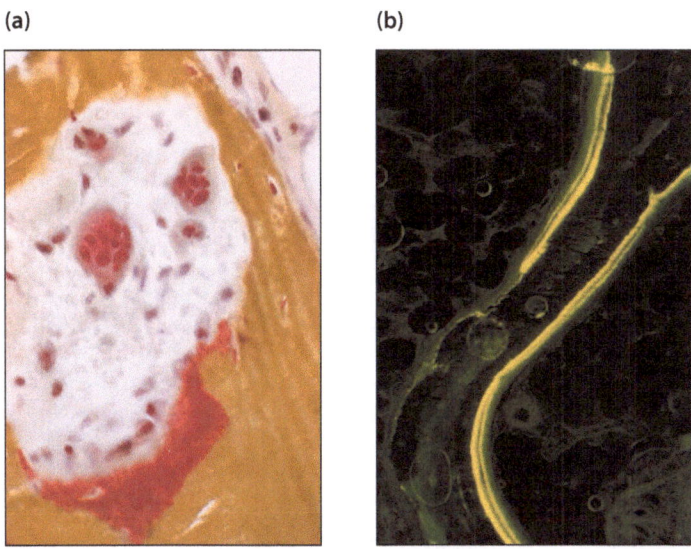

MicroCT image of transiliac bone biopsies taken in postmenopausal osteoporotic women

Figure 3.20. Quantitative microcomputed tomography (microCT) image of human biopsies using a Scanco 40 instrument allows a three-dimensional approach of the microarchitecture. In particular, it allows the form of the trabeculae (plates or rods) to be evaluated, which is important in determining the mechanical properties of the trabecular bone and represents a clear advantage over classical histomorphometry. In this figure, transiliac bone biopsies taken in postmenopausal osteoporotic women show that the trabecular microarchitecture is better following 3 years of treatment with strontium ranelate 2 g/day (right) than with placebo (left). Adapted from Arlot M, Jiang Y, Genant HK et al. Histomorphometric and μCT analysis of bone biopsies from postmenopausal osteoporotic women treated with strontium ranelate. J Bone Miner Res 2008, 23:215–22.

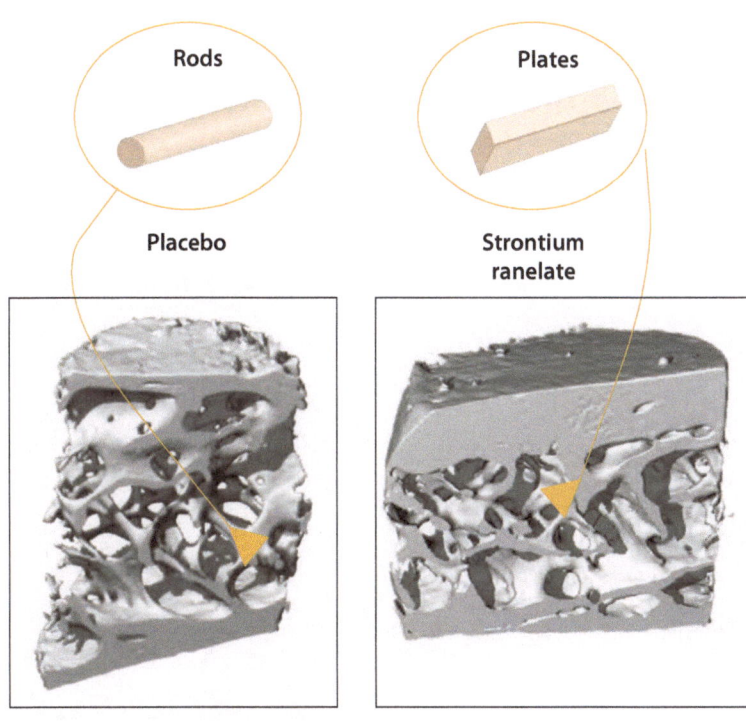

In vivo microCT with an Xtreme CT scanner

Figure 3.21. (a) Xtreme CT scanner. **(b)** *In vivo* high resolution peripheral quantitative computed tomography (HR-pQCT) image of a sagittal section of a human tibia (left) and radius (right). This technique is noninvasive and provides a three-dimensional reconstruction of bone with a resolution of 82 μm *in vivo*. Reproduced with permission from Boutroy S, Bouxsein ML, Munoz F et al. In vivo assessment of trabecular bone microarchitecture by high-resolution peripheral quantitative computed tomography. J Clin Endocrinol Metab 2005; 90:6508–15.

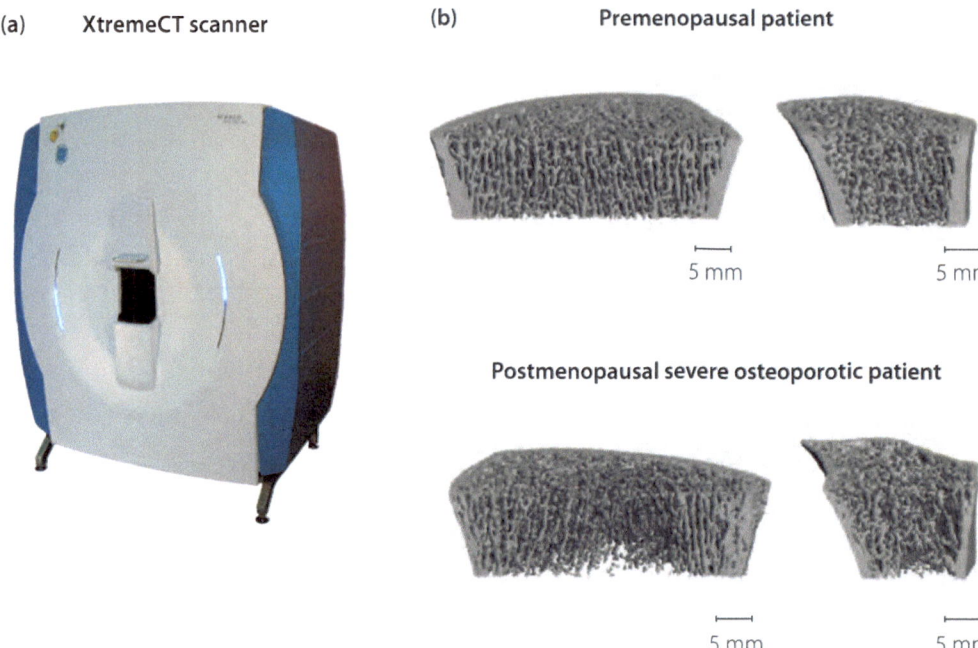

(a) XtremeCT scanner

(b) Premenopausal patient

5 mm 5 mm

Postmenopausal severe osteoporotic patient

5 mm 5 mm

The importance of bone microarchitecture

Figure 3.22. The supportive strength of a series of columns can be greatly enhanced, but with a minimal effect on mass, by adding a few relatively small cross-struts. Similarly, in bone a small increase in the mass of structurally important trabeculae has little effect on bone mineral density but improves bone strength greatly. In osteoporosis the thinning of these cross-struts, or trabeculae, greatly decreases bone strength. This thinning can be seen on the accompanying microscopic images of normal and osteoporotic bone. Images courtesy of J Kosek, Stanford University School of Medicine, Stanford, California, USA.

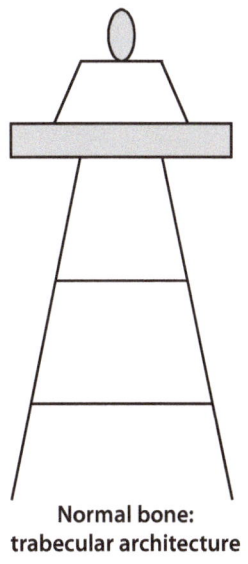

**Normal bone:
trabecular architecture**

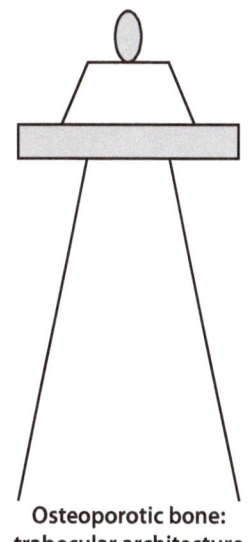

**Osteoporotic bone:
trabecular architecture**

Load resistance:

180 kg

20 kg

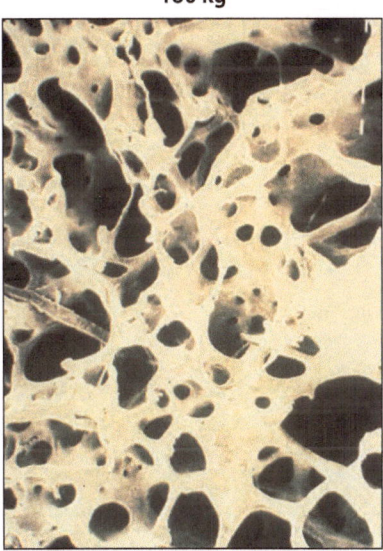

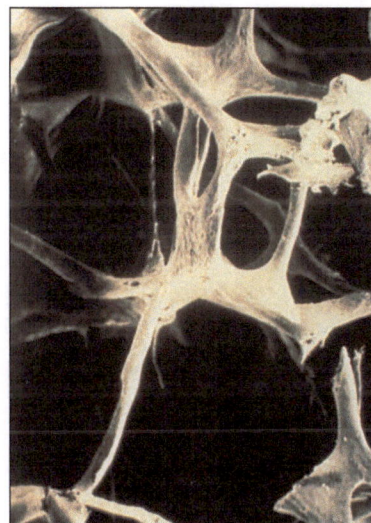

Degree of mineralization

Figure 3.23. Effect of alendronate on the distribution of the degree of mineralization measured in compact bone of ovariectomized baboons. In ovariectomized animals treated with alendronate, the degree of bone mineralization (1.196 g mineral/cm^3 bone) was higher than that of the untreated ovariectomized baboon (0.716 g mineral/cm^3 bone) but was similar to that of the control baboons (1.254 g mineral/cm^3 bone). Reproduced with permission from Meunier PJ, Boivin G. Bone mineral density reflects bone mass but also degree of mineralization of bone: therapeutic implications. Bone 1997; 21:373–7.

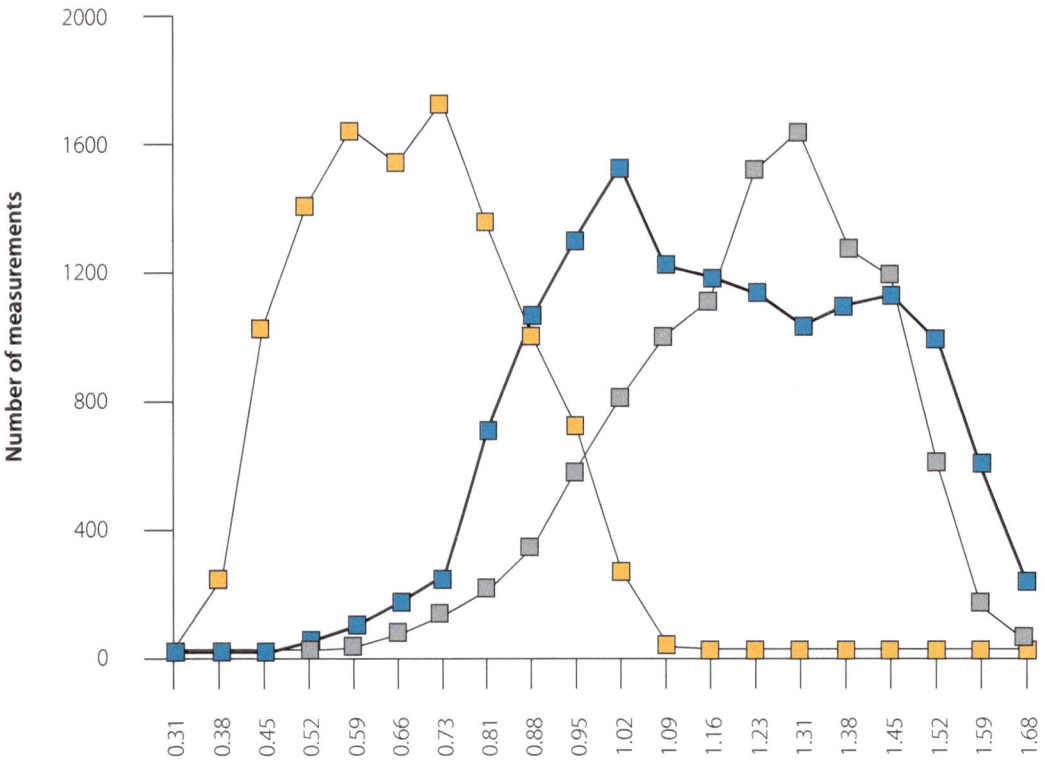

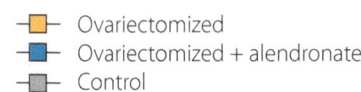

Effects of alendronate in compact bone

Figure 3.24. Microradiographs of compact bone from the tibia of control baboons (CTRL), ovariectomized animals (OVX), and ovariectomized baboons treated with alendronate (ALN). The images show the variations in the degree of mineralization induced by the changes in bone remodeling activity (original magnification ×35). Fully mineralized tissue is white and tissue still undergoing mineralization is gray. Reproduced with permission from Meunier PJ, Boivin G. Bone mineral density reflects bone mass but also degree of mineralization of bone: therapeutical implications. Bone 1997; 21:373–7.

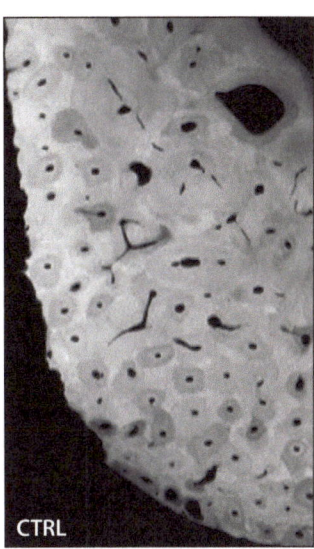 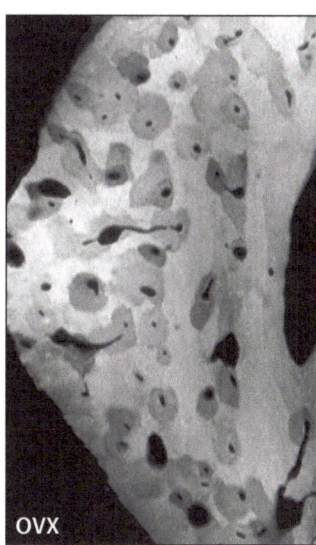 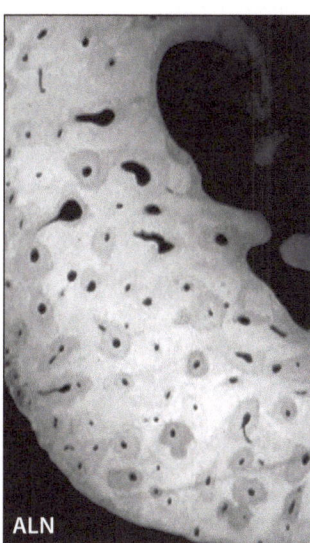

Rate of bone remodeling and bone strength

Figure 3.25. The rate of bone remodeling is a determinant of bone strength. This schematic representation shows the normal bone remodeling (SHAM), after ovariectomy (OVX), and in OVX rats treated with bisphosphonates. The mineralized bone is represented in blue and bone in a phase of remodeling in white. The arrows represent the forces exerted. By changing the distribution of stress in relation to the volume of bone in a phase of remodeling, a high remodeling rate may decrease mechanical strength. Depending on the amount of bone under remodeling, a given force is distributed among different volumes of bone. From Ammann P, Rizzoli R. Bone strength and its determinants. Osteoporos Int 2003; 14(Suppl 3):S13–S18.

SHAM   OVX   OVX + bisphosphonate

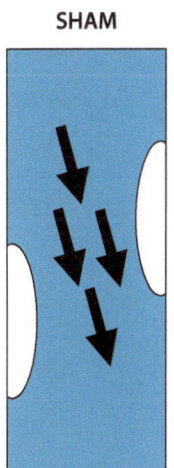 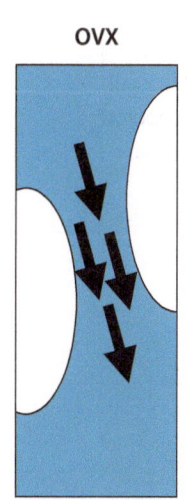 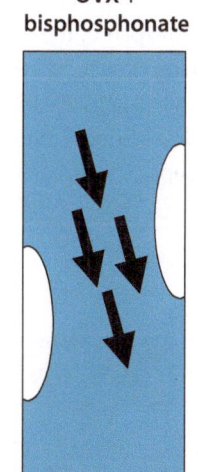

Intrinsic bone quality: trabecular/cortical nanoindentation

Figure 3.26. The nanoindentation technique is used to investigate tissue quality by measuring both hardness and elasticity of dry and wet bone tissue with a high spatial resolution. Nanoindentation testing involves compressing a pyramidal diamond tip into a material, and simultaneously recording force and displacement with milli-Newton and nanometer resolution. From the resulting force–displacement curves, hardness (the maximal force per unit area) and indentation modulus (a purely elastic property) can be calculated. The nanoindentation method allows the mechanical properties of single bone structural units to be quantified. Nanoindentation testing has the potential to become a major new tool in the assessment of bone quality, and elucidation of mechanisms by which treatments for osteoporosis improve bone strength. Adapted from Zysset PK, Guo XE, Hoffler CE et al. Elastic modulus and hardness of cortical and trabecular bone lamellae measured by nanoindentation in the human femur. J Biomech 1999; 32:1005–12.

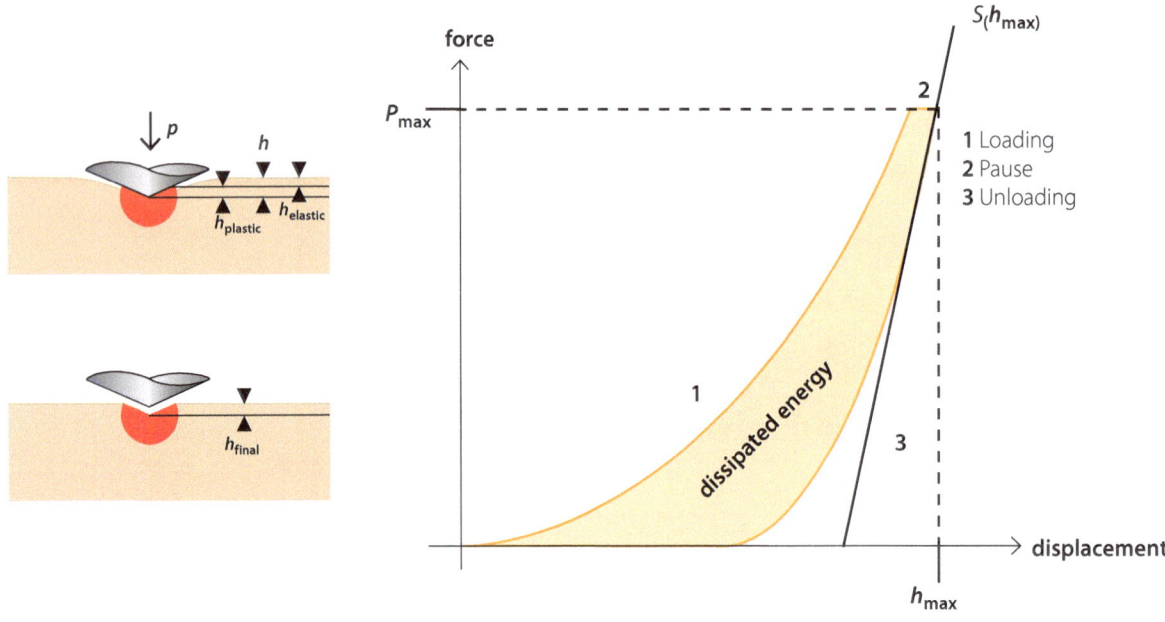

Axial compression and three-point bending tests

Figure 3.27. Evaluation of bone strength in different parts of the skeleton: **(a)** compression of the vertebral body or of proximal tibia, and **(b)** three-point bending test of the long bones, such as tibia, femur, or humerus. The tests are performed at different skeletal sites characterized by various proportions of cortical and trabecular bone. In order to take into account all the determinants of bone strength, the integrity of the investigated bone sample should be preserved. To preserve integrity of intact vertebrae embedding the plateaux of the intact vertebrae in methylmethacrylate allows a uniform distribution of the stresses on the bone specimen, and is preferable to sawing of the proximal and distal part of the vertebral body. Attention must also be paid to testing a weight-bearing structure containing large proportions of trabecular bone, for example, using compression tests of the proximal tibia, as this site is sensitive to antiosteoporotic treatments. For each of these tests a load–deflection curve is generated (see Figure 3.29). From Ammann P, Rizzoli R. Bone strength and its determinants. Osteoporos Int 2003; 14(Suppl 3):S13–S18.

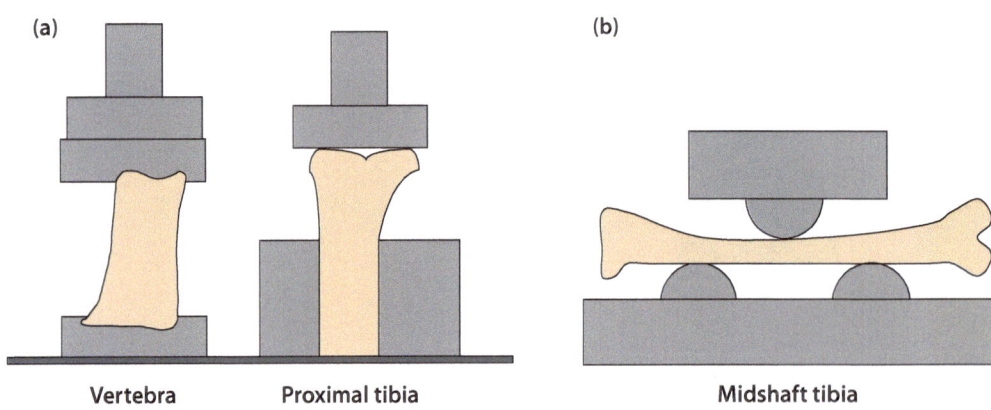

Compression test of vertebra (L4)

Figure 3.28. Strontium ranelate treatment is associated with a significant increase in plastic energy (yellow). This corresponds to an increased capacity of bone tissue to accomodate microdamage before fracture, which represents an improvement of bone tissue quality. The distance between the two horizontal lines (indicated by arrows) corresponds to the influence of strontium ranelate on bone strength. Adapted from Ammann P, Badoud I, Barraud S et al. Strontium ranelate treatment improves trabecular and cortical intrinsic bone tissue quality, a determinant of bone strength. J Bone Miner Res 2007: 22:1419–25.

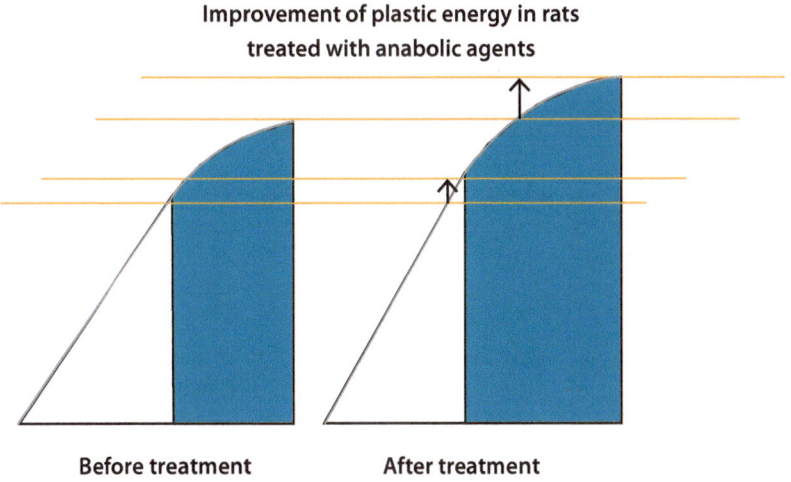

Improvement of plastic energy in rats treated with anabolic agents

Before treatment　　　　After treatment

Load–deflection curve

Figure 3.29. A load–deflection curve can be recorded, enabling calculation of various components: stiffness, by measuring the slope of the linear part of the curve; ultimate strength, by measuring the highest load obtained before fracture; and energy absorbed (toughness) at maximal load, by measuring the area under the curve. Other parameters can be derived, for example, the yield point, which corresponds to the transition from an elastic to a plastic, or irreversible deformation of the sample. Adapted from Jørgensen RH, Bak B, Andressen TT. Mechanical properties and biochemical composition of rat cortical femur and tibia after long-term treatment with biosynthetic human growth hormone. Bone 1991; 12:353–9.

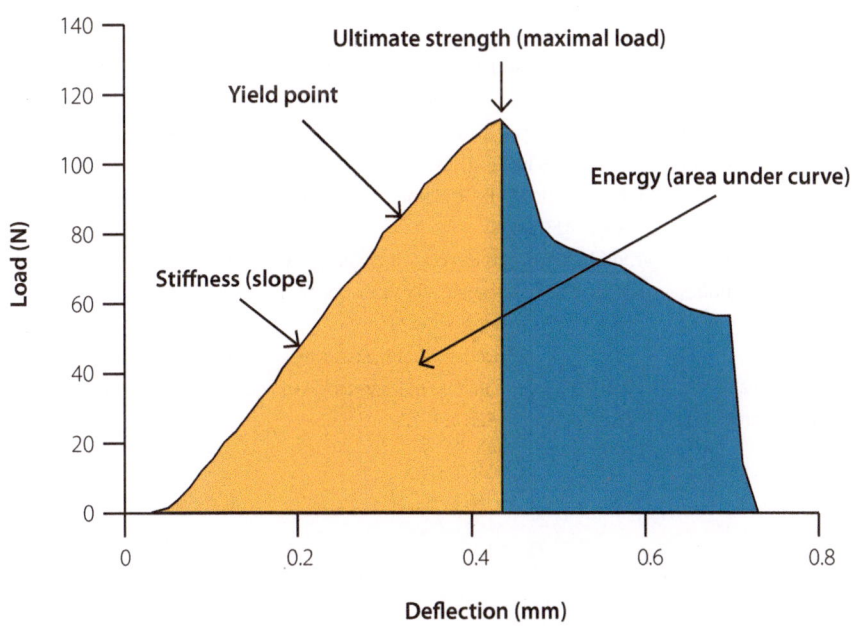

References

Ammann P, Badoud I, Barraud S, et al. Strontium ranelate treatment improves trabecular and cortical intrinsic bone tissue quality, a determinant of bone strength. J Bone Miner Res 2007: 22:1419–25.

Ammann P, Bourrin S, Bonjour JP et al. Protein undernutritioninduced bone loss is associated with decreased IGF-1 levels and estrogen deficiency. J Bone Miner Res 2000; 15:683–90.

Ammann P, Laib A, Bonjour JP et al. Dietary essential amino acid supplements increase bone strength by influencing bone mass and bone microarchitecture in ovariectomized adult rats fed an isocaloric low-protein diet. J Bone Min Res 2002; 17:1264–72.

Ammann P, Rizzoli R. Bone strength and its determinants. Osteoporos Int 2003; 14(Suppl 3):S13–S18.

Ammann P, Rizzoli R, Bonjour JP. Preclinical evaluation of new therapeutic agents for osteoporosis. In: Osteoporosis: Diagnosis and Management. Edited by PJ Meunier. London: Martin Dunitz, 1998; 257–73.

Ammann P, Rizzoli R, Meyer JM et al. Bone density and shape as determinants of bone strength in IGF-1 and/or pamidronate-treated ovariectomized rats. Osteoporos Int 1996; 6:219–27.

Ammann P, Shen V, Robin B et al. Strontium ranelate improves bone resistance by increasing bone mass and improving architecture in intact female rats. Bone Miner Res 2004; 19:2012–20.

Andreassen TT, Jorgensen PH, Flyvbjerg A et al. Growth hormone stimulates bone formation and strength of cortical bone in aged rats. J Bone Miner Res 1995; 10:1057–67.

Arlot M, Jiang Y, Genant HK, et al. Histomorphometric and µCT analysis of bone biopsies from postmenopausal osteoporotic women treated with strontium ranelate. J Bone Miner Res 2008, 23:215–222.

Bagi CM, Ammann P, Rizzoli R et al. Effect of estrogen deficiency on cancellous and cortical bone structure and strength of the femoral neck in rats. Calcif Tissue Int 1997; 61:336–44.

Bain SD, Jerome C, Shen I, et al. Strontium ranelate improves bone strength in ovariectomized rat by positively influencing bone resistance determinants. Osteoporosis Int 2009; 20:1417–28.

Boivin GY, Chavassieux PM, Santora AC et al. Alendronate increases bone strength by increasing the mean degree of mineralization of bone tissue in osteoporotic women. Bone 2000; 27:687–94.

Boivin G, Meunier PJ. Changes in bone remodeling rate influence the degree of mineralization of bone which is a determinant of bone strength: therapeutic implications. Adv Exp Med Biol 2001; 496:123–7.

Bonjour JP, Ammann P, Rizzoli R. Importance of preclinical studies in the development of drugs for treatment of osteoporosis: a review related to the 1998 WHO guidelines. Osteoporos Int 1999; 9:379–93.

Bourrin S, Ammann P, Bonjour JP et al. Recovery of proximal tibia bone mineral density and strength, but not cancellous bone architecture, after long-term bisphosphonate or selective estrogen receptor modulator therapy in aged rats. Bone 2002; 30:195–200.

Bourrin S, Ammann P, Bonjour JP et al. Dietary protein restriction lowers plasma insulin-like growth factor 1 (IGF-1), impairs cortical bone formation, and induces osteoblastic resistance to IGF-1 in adult female rats. Endocrinology 2000; 141:3149–55.

Boutroy S, Bouxsein ML, Munoz F et al. In vivo assessment of trabecular bone microarchitecture by high-resolution peripheral quantitative computed tomography. J Clin Endocrinol Metab 2005; 90:6508–15.

Bouxsein ML, Coan BS, Lee SC. Prediction of the strength of the elderly proximal femur by bone mineral density and quantitative ultrasound measurements of the heel and tibia. Bone 1999; 25:49–54.

Brennan TC, Rizzoli R, Ammann P. Selective modification of bone quality by PTH, pamidronate or raloxifene. J Bone Miner Res 2009; 24:800–8.

Chavassieux PM, Arlot ME, Reda C et al. Histomorphometric assessment of the long-term effects of alendronate on bone quality and remodeling in patients with osteoporosis. J Clin Invest 1997; 100:1475–80.

Delmas P, San Martin J, Chen P et al. Severity of vertebral fracture reflects deterioration of trabecular bone microarchictecture. Osteoporos Int 2005; 16:319.

Ejersted C, Andreassen TT, Oxlund H et al. Human parathyroid hormone (1–34) and (1–84) increase the mechanical strength and thickness of cortical bone in rats. J Bone Miner Res 1993; 8:1097–101.

Garnero P, Hausherr E, Chapuy MC et al. Markers of bone resorption predict hip fracture in elderly women: the EPIDOS Prospective Study. J Bone Miner Res 1996; 11:1531–8.

Granhed H, Jonson R, Hansson T. Mineral content and strength of lumbar vertebrae. A cadaver study. Acta Orthop Scand 1989; 60:105–9.

Hauselmann HJ, Rizzoli R. A comprehensive review of treatments for postmenopausal osteoporosis. Osteoporos Int 2003; 14:2–12.

Hengsberger S, Ammann P, Legros B et al. Intrinsic bone tissue properties in adult rat vertebrae: modulation by dietary protein. Bone 2005; 36:134–41.

Hoffler CE, Moore KE, Kozloff K et al. Age, gender, and bone lamellae elastic moduli. J Orthop Res 2000; 18:432–27.

Jørgensen PH, Bak B, Andreassen TT. Mechanical properties and biochemical composition of rat cortical femur and tibia after long-term treatment with biosynthetic human growth hormone. Bone 1991; 12:353–9.

Mashiba T, Turner CH, Hirano T et al. Effects of suppressed bone turnover by bisphosphonates on microdamage accumulation and biomechanical properties in clinically relevant skeletal sites in Beagles. Bone 2001; 28:524–31.

Meunier PJ, Boivin G. Bone mineral density reflects bone mass but also degree of mineralization of bone: therapeutical implications. Bone 1997; 21:373–7.

Parfitt AM, Drezner MK, Glorieux FH et al. Bone histomorphometry: standardization of nomenclature, symbols and units. J Bone Miner Res 1987; 2:595–610.

Rho J, Tsui T, Pharr O. Elastic properties of human cortical and trabecular lamellar bone measured by nanoindentation. Biomaterials 1997; 18:1325–30.

Riggs BL, Melton LJ 3rd. Bone turnover matters: the raloxifene treatment paradox of dramatic decreases in vertebral fractures without commensurate increases in bone density. J Bone Miner Res 2002; 17:11–4.

Turner CH. Biomechanics of bone: determinants of skeletal fragility and bone quality. Osteoporos Int 2002; 13:97–104.

Turner CH. Toward a cure for osteoporosis: reversal of excessive bone fragility. Osteoporos Int 1991; 2:12–9.

Turner CH, Burr DB. Basic biomechanical measurements of bone: a tutorial. Bone 1993; 14:595–608.

World Health Organization Study Group. Assessment of fracture risk and its application to screening for postmenopausal osteoporosis. World Health Organ Tech Rep Ser 1994; 843:1–129.

Zysset PK, Guo XE, Hoffler CE et al. Elastic modulus and hardness of cortical and trabecular bone lamellae measured by nanoindentation in the human femur. J Biomech 1999; 32:1005–12.

Chapter 4

Prevention and treatment of postmenopausal osteoporosis

Audrey Neuprez and Jean-Yves Reginster

Due to the high personal and societal costs of osteoporosis, the condition remains a challenge to both public health and physicians [Kanis et al. 2008]. Furthermore, the rapid increase in the elderly population means that the prevention of osteoporotic fracture is a socioeconomic priority [Suzuki et al. 2008].

However, the majority of postmenopausal osteoporosis patients remain untreated [Kanis et al. 2008], and even treatment-compliant patients experience new vertebral or nonvertebral fragility fractures during therapy at a rate of 9.5% per year [Adami et al. 2009], leaving a significant proportion of effectively treated patients at risk of fracture. It has also been observed that just 6% of previously untreated patients hospitalized for hip fracture are prescribed antiosteoporotic therapy, with only 41% persisting with treatment at 12 months, at a median duration of 40.3 weeks [Rabenda et al. 2008]. Consequently, it is crucial that effective management strategies are developed.

Despite the fact that postmenopausal osteoporotic fractures are most common in women over 65 years of age, and interventions have only been shown to be effective in populations with an average age over 65 years, most of the available interventions nevertheless prevent, slow, or reverse bone loss when started at around 50 years of age. It is, therefore, advisable to begin identifying patients from this age who have osteoporosis or who are at risk of developing this condition [Kanis et al. 2008].

Goals of intervention

The clinical significance of postmenopausal osteoporosis results from the fractures that arise. The principal aim of preventing and treating postmenopausal osteoporosis is therefore to reduce the frequency of fragility fractures (Figure 4.1) [Adami et al. 2009], which are largely responsible for the morbidity and, indirectly, the mortality related to the condition [Delmas, 2002].

Poor adherence is a continuing problem in postmenopausal osteoporosis management, reducing the potential efficacy of treatment [Kanis et al. 2008]. Factors associated with adherence include belief in the importance of taking medications, medication-specific factors such as administration requirements, beliefs regarding medications and health, relationships with healthcare providers, the exchange of information, and strategies to improve adherence, which include systems for taking medications, cues or reminders to take the medication, knowledge of the reasons for taking the medication, and regular follow-up and monitoring [Lau et al. 2008].

Nonpharmacological approaches

Various nonpharmacological measures can reduce the risk of developing postmenopausal osteoporosis, which, in general, should be recommended to all women, including adequate exercise, a diet rich in calcium, stopping smoking, and avoiding excessive alcohol intake (Figure 4.2).

Exercise

Regular physical exercise is thought to reduce the risk of osteoporosis, and delay the physiologic decrease of bone mineral density (BMD) that occurs with ageing [Ernst, 1998]. In addition, immobilization is an important cause of bone loss, leading to as much lost in a week as could be expected to be lost in a year [Kanis et al. 2008]. High-charge exercises have been shown to increase the BMD of the spinal column and high-intensity exercises to increase bone density at the hip and forearm, and other types of exercise may be helpful [Banciu et al. 2005] (Figure 4.3). While the optimal amount of weight-bearing exercise for osteoporosis patients is unknown, increased strength may improve confidence and coordination as well as maintain bone mass by stimulating bone formation and by decreasing bone resorption [Kanis et al. 2008].

Diet

Elderly patients have a high prevalence of calcium, protein, and vitamin D insufficiency [Kanis et al. 2008]. It is widely believed that a poor dietary intake of calcium is a risk factor for osteoporosis (Figure 4.4); however, other nutrients are needed to maintain healthy bone. High dietary levels of phosphates (found for example in many carbonated drinks) are associated with a negative calcium balance [Mundy, 2001]. Sufficient protein intake is required to maintain the integrity and function of the musculoskeletal system, in addition to which it decreases the complications resulting from osteoporotic fracture [Kanis et al. 2008]. This improves the clinical course of hip fracture, as well as shortening the duration of hospital stay [Kanis et al. 2008]. European guidelines recommend a daily protein intake of at least 1 g/kg body weight. Eating disorders, such as anorexia nervosa, are associated with later osteoporosis, owing, in part, at least, to reduced body weight [Hotta, 1998]. Certainly, a well-balanced diet should be recommended for women of all ages.

Fall prevention

Most fractures other than vertebral fractures are associated with falls. This is true in the general population as well as among postmenopausal women. Falls increase with impaired mobility/disability, impaired gait and balance, neuromuscular or musculoskeletal disorders, age, impaired vision, neurological and heart disorders, history of falls, medication, and cognitive impairment [Kanis et al. 2008]. Moreover, the risk of injury from any single fall increases with age [Wehren, 2003]. Women start to fall more frequently by approximately 50 years of age. By the age of 70 years, some 20% of women fall at least once a year; by the age of 80 years, this figure has risen to 48% [Winner et al. 1989]. It follows then that prevention of falls is likely to reduce the incidence of fractures in elderly women. The home environment may be improved by reducing slippery floors, obstacles, and insufficient lighting, and installing handrails [Kanis et al. 2008] However, while the risk of falls is reduced, the risk of fracture is not significantly reduced [Kanis et al. 2008]. The use of hip protectors has been found to be effective in reducing the incidence of hip fractures when they are worn (Figure 4.5). There is, however, poor compliance with hip protectors because of discomfort and impracticality, and recent meta-analyses have called into question their antifracture efficacy [Kanis et al. 2008].

Smoking cessation

Smoking increases bone loss. It has been shown to have a significant impact on femoral neck BMD, and lumbar spine BMD [Hansen et al. 1991; Egger et al. 1996]. One study of elderly patients found that each decade of smoking reduces femoral neck BMD by an average of 0.011 g/cm^2, and lumbar spine BMD by an average of 0.015 g/cm^2 [Egger et al. 1996]. Smoking has been estimated to increase the overall lifetime risk of a woman developing a vertebral fracture by 13%, and a hip fracture by 31%. Moreover, smoking appears to reduce the beneficial effects on bone of postmenopausal hormone replacement therapy [Kiel, 1992]. Smoking cessation may have a positive effect on BMD [Ward & Klesges, 2001].

Pharmacological approaches

Antiresorptive agents

Calcium and vitamin D

Many studies have investigated the effect of vitamin D and calcium supplements on osteoporosis and fracture risk in postmenopausal women.

In order to address this question it is necessary to consider threshold intakes of vitamin D and calcium below which skeletal health is compromised. Ideally, this should be based on the establishment of the relationship between nutrient intake and a measurable index of skeletal health. For vitamin D it is possible to determine a plausible threshold in that many studies have characterised a relationship between low circulating levels of 25-hydroxyvitamin D (25[OH]D) and increased secretion of parathyroid hormone (PTH) which in turn, induces bone loss in the elderly through increased bone resorption [Boonen et al. 2007; Chapuy et al. 2002; Sahota et al. 2004].

Published estimates of the level of circulating 25(OH)D required to maintain normal levels of PTH range between 30 and 100 nmol/l [Dawson-Hughes et al. 2005]. This in turn means that estimates of vitamin D insufficiency within populations vary greatly depending on the threshold used. In a study of 8532 postmenopausal, osteoporotic European women, 79.6% were found to have vitamin D insufficiency where the serum 25(OH)D threshold was considered to be 80 nmol/l, and 32.1% if the threshold was set at 50 nmol/l [Bruyère et al. 2006]. In one study, PTH fell by 35% in subjects with baseline 25(OH)D levels between 27.5 and 39.9 nmol/l after 8 weeks of supplementation, by 26% in those with levels between 40 and 49.9 nmol/l, but there was no significant change in PTH in those with 25(OH)D levels superior to 50 nmol/l, despite a 66% increase in the vitamin D metabolite [Malabanan et al. 1998]. After discussion of current evidence it was agreed by a European panel that 80 nmol/l may be an overestimate and that 50 nmol/l was a more conservative and acceptable threshold [Rizzoli et al. 2008a].

Vitamin D supplementation must be sufficient to ensure that serum 25(OH)D values reach the threshold level, otherwise it will not confer the desired benefit. Studies investigating the antifracture efficacy of different dosing regimens of vitamin D have shown that 400 IU per day was not sufficient to have an effect on fracture rate [Bischoff-Ferrari et al. 2005]. Oral doses of > 700–800 IU taken daily or 100,000 IU taken quarterly both showed a positive antifracture effect, whereas an intramuscular dose of 300,000 IU annually showed inconsistent efficacy [Bischoff-Ferrari et al. 2005; Heikinheimo et al. 1992]. This suggests that supplementation is most effective in osteoporotic patients if given orally either daily or quarterly, and if given daily, should be in excess of 700–800 IU daily [Bischoff-Ferrari, 2007]. The situation regarding an acceptable threshold for dietary calcium intake is far less clear, and recommendations range from 400 to 1500 mg daily [Rizzoli et al. 2008a].

Current evidence suggests the role that calcium and vitamin D play in fracture prevention is not attributable to calcium alone [Prince et al. 2006; Shea et al. 2002] and a meta-analysis of data from nine randomized clinical trials, including a total of 53,260 patients, found that where the effects of supplementation with vitamin D alone were explored (in a total of 9038 patients), this was not sufficient to significantly reduce the risk of hip fracture in postmenopausal women [Boonen et al. 2007]. However the same study found that combined supplementation with vitamin D and calcium reduced the risk of hip fracture by 25% (95% CI: 4–42) and the risk of nonvertebral fracture by 23% (95% CI: 1–40) compared with supplementation with vitamin D alone. The meta-analysis estimated the number needed to treat (NNT) to prevent one adverse outcome to be 276 (95% CI: 165–843) for hip fractures and 72 (95% CI: 35–834) for nonvertebral fractures .

These results support a previous meta-analysis which has shown a reduction of 19% (95% CI: 4–32) for hip fracture and of 13% (95% CI: 3–22) for any nonvertebral fracture [Avenell et al. 2005].

Compliance in the various trials could explain the difference in the number needed to treat reported in 2 recent meta-analyses, one including mainly high quality randomized controlled trials [Bischoff-Ferrari et al. 2005] and the other one including additional studies with lower compliance, such as the RECORD and WHI trials. In the former meta-analysis, NNT was 45 (95% CI: 28–114) and 27 (95% CI: 19–49), for hip and any nonvertebral fracture, respectively.

Given the low cost of vitamin D and calcium supplements, compared with the high economic burden of osteoporotic fractures, combined supplementation can be economically justified.

In order to reduce fracture risk, combined supplementation should be administered to those at increased risk of fracture at doses adjusted depending on baseline levels, but potentially in the region of 800 IU of vitamin D and 1000–1200 mg of calcium daily.

The vast majority of evidence for efficacy of antiosteoporotic treatments is based upon combining treatment with calcium and vitamin D supplementation [Bone et al. 2004; Neer et al. 2001; Harris et al. 1999; Ettinger et al. 1999; Chesnut et al. 2000; Meunier et al. 2004; Delmas, 2002]. Vitamin D deficiency in humans and animals has been shown to reduce the response to some treatments for osteoporosis. In addition, animal studies have shown that the efficacy of bisphosphonates was blunted when the animals were exposed to a vitamin D deprived diet [Mastaglia et al. 2006] It is concluded therefore that antiosteoporotic treatments should be used in combination with calcium and vitamin D supplementation. Little evidence is available regarding the combination of antiosteoporotic treatments with calcium alone or vitamin D alone.

Hormone replacement therapy

Estrogen deficiency has long been known to be associated with osteoporosis, and estrogen replacement has been considered the gold standard for its prevention [Eastell, 1998]. It has a consistently beneficial effect on BMD at all sites. It has also been reported to reduce the relative risk of fracture of the spine by up to 50% and nonvertebral fractures by approximately 30% (Figure 4.6) [Cauley, 2003; Torgerson & Bell-Syer, 2001a; 2001b]. For many years hormone replacement therapy (HRT) was used as the first-line therapy in the prevention of postmenopausal osteoporosis, with its most beneficial effects being seen when it was started early during the menopausal period. Two recent large studies, the Women's Health Initiative Study, and the Million Women Study, have, however, confirmed that the use of HRT is associated with increased risks of breast cancer and cardiovascular disease [Beral, 2003; Rossouw, 2002]. Patients are now advised to use HRT for the shortest time possible, at as low a dose as possible in order to stop the menopausal symptoms, such as flushes, and only when benefits outweigh the risks (eg, in symptomatic menopausal women). It is, therefore, not a valid option for the long-term prevention of fracture, and there is a need to find alternatives to the use of HRT in healthy postmenopausal women in order to prevent osteoporosis.

Tibolone

Tibolone is a synthetic, non-estrogen steroid. Its metabolites may have estrogenic, androgenic, and progestogenic properties, depending on its tissue of activity. It has been shown to increase the BMD of trabecular bone, without a simultaneous loss of cortical bone, and to reduce bone turnover. These effects are thought to be due to an estrogenic effect, although there may be an androgenic effect as well [Rubin & Bilezikian, 2003]. A placebo-controlled study demonstrated that, over a median treatment period of 34 months, tibolone 1.25 mg once daily increases BMD by 4.8% in the spine and 3.1% in the femoral neck [Cummings et al. 2008]. In addition, the results showed that tibolone reduces the risk of vertebral and nonvertebral fracture, at relative hazard ratios of 0.55 and 0.74, respectively [Cummings et al. 2008]. While tibolone also decreased the risk of invasive breast cancer and colon cancer, at respective relative hazard ratios of 0.32 and 0.31, the risk of stroke was increased, at a relative hazard ratio of 2.19, causing the trial to be halted [Cummings et al. 2008].

Selective estrogen receptor modulators

The selective estrogen receptor modulators (SERMs) are non-steroidal agents that bind to the estrogen receptor (Figure 4.7). They exert an estrogenic effect in some target tissues, such as bone, but not in others, thus reducing the rate of bone loss, and making them an alternative to estrogen therapy in postmenopausal osteoporosis (Figure 4.8). Raloxifene, a benzothiophene, is the only SERM used today for the management of osteoporosis, but several others are in clinical development [Kanis et al. 2008]. Raloxifene has been shown to increase BMD (Figure 4.9), with the effect increasing over 2 years. In a large phase III clinical trial among women with osteoporosis, as defined by a low BMD or radiographic vertebral fractures, raloxifene was shown to increase bone density, and reduce the incidence of vertebral fractures in patients with and without prevalent vertebral fractures (Figure 4.10). Raloxifene does not, however, have a significant effect on nonvertebral fractures, except in patients with severe vertebral fractures at baseline [Delmas et al. 2003; Barrett-Connor et al. 2002; Ettinger et al. 1999; Delmas et al. 1997]. Raloxifene decreases the risk of breast cancer by approximately 60%, which has been confirmed for up to 8 years of treatment [Martino et al. 2004]. The benzothiophene is taken as a once-daily tablet and can increase hot flushes. It also increases the risk of venous thrombo-embolic disease, but not the risk of cardiovascular disease.

Bisphosphonates

Bisphosphonates are stable pyrophosphate analogs with a P–C–P bond [Kanis et al. 2008] (Figure 4.11). A range of bisphosphonates have been synthesized, and their potency depends on the length and structure of the side chain, ranging 10,000-fold *in vitro*. They have a strong affinity for bone apatite. They inhibit bone resorption reducing the recruitment and activity of osteoclasts, and increasing their apoptosis [Watts, 2003]. The mechanism includes inhibition of the proton vacuolar adenosine triphosphatease and alteration of the cytoskeleton and ruffled border. In addition, nitrogen-containing bisphosphonates interfere with the mevalonate pathway and protein prenylation (Figure 4.12). The oral bioavailability of bisphosphonates is low, at 1–3% of the ingested dose, and is impaired by food, calcium, iron, coffee, tea, and orange juice. Approximately 50% of bisphosphonates in the plasma are deposited in bone and the rest is excreted in urine. However, they have a long half-life [Kanis et al. 2008].

The bisphosphonates increase BMD in early postmenopausal women, thus preventing the development of osteoporosis [Cranney et al. 2002a; 2002b]. Bisphosphonates are considered as a first-line therapy for the treatment of postmenopausal osteoporosis [Brown & Josse, 2002]. Bisphosphonates increase BMD in those with established osteoporosis and reduce the risk of vertebral fracture. A cost-effectiveness analysis indicated that bisphosphonates increase treatment costs by 21%, but decrease the number of fractures by 35%, with the additional cost of therapy offset by other cost savings if the treatment is targeted at high-risk women [Tosteson et al. 2008].

The most commonly used bisphosphonates are alendronate 70 mg once weekly and risedronate 35 mg once weekly. In a phase III clinical trial of postmenopausal women with low bone mass with vertebral fractures, alendronate was shown to reduce the frequency of vertebral and of some nonvertebral fractures (ie, hip and wrist) (Figure 4.13). In those without vertebral fractures, alendronate increased BMD (Figure 4.14). While it failed to reduce the risk of clinical fractures overall, the reduction was significant among women with low baseline hip BMD T-scores. [Cummings et al. 1998; Black et al. 1996]. A 12-week, placebo-controlled trial showed that alendronate 20 mg once-weekly significantly reduced the bone resorption markers serum bone-specific alkaline phosphatase (BSAP), osteocalcin, and C-terminal telopeptide of type 1 collagen (CTX) [Choi et al. 2008].

Risedronate has been shown to increase BMD at the spine and hip, and reduce the incidence of new vertebral and nonvertebral fractures in women with established osteoporosis by 40–50% and 30–39%, respectively (Figure 4.15) [Reginster et al. 2000; Harris et al. 1999]. It also reduces the risk of hip fractures in elderly women by 30% (Figure 4.16) [McClung et al. 2001] and the risk of vertebral fractures in patients over 80 years of age [Boonen et al. 2004]. A 2-year comparison trial of alendronate 70 mg once weekly and risedronate 35 mg once weekly revealed that postmenopausal osteoporotic women experience significantly greater increases in BMD at the hip trochanter, total hip, femoral neck, and lumbar spine, at treatment differences of 1.0–1.7% [Reid et al. 2008]. Alendronate also causes significantly larger decreases in the four markers of bone turnover N-telopeptide of type 1 human collagen, CTX, BSAP, and serum N-terminal propeptide of type 1 procollagen (PINP).

The incidence of hip and nonvertebral fractures among women in the year following initiation of once-a-week dosing of either risedronate or alendronate was observed using records of health service utilization. Through 1 year of therapy, the incidence of nonvertebral fractures in the risedronate cohort (2.0%) was 18% lower (95% CI 2–32%) than in the alendronate cohort (2.3%). The incidence of hip fractures in the risedronate cohort (0.4%) was 43% lower (95% CI 13–63%) than in the alendronate cohort (0.6%) [Silverman et al. 2007].

Ibandronate 2.5 mg daily reduces the risk of vertebral fractures by 50–60% (Figure 4.17). However, ibandronate has an effect on nonvertebral fractures only in women with a low baseline BMD T-score [Delmas et al. 2004]. Bridging studies have shown that oral ibandronate 150 mg once monthly is equivalent or superior to daily ibandronate in increasing BMD and decreasing biochemical markers of bone turnover, giving rise to its approval for the treatment of postmenopausal osteoporosis [Reginster et al. 2006]. Another investigation revealed that ibandronate 150 mg once monthly improves vertebral, peripheral, and trabecular strength and anteroposterior bending stiffness compared with placebo, at 7.1%, 7.8%, 5.6%, and 6.3%, respectively, along with femoral narrow neck cross-sectional area and outer diameter, at 3.6% and 2.2%, respectively [Lewiecki et al. 2009].

Similarly, bridging studies comparing intermittent intravenous ibandronate with daily oral treatment has lead to the approval of intravenous ibandronate (3 mg) every 3 months for the treatment of postmenopausal osteoporosis [Delmas et al. 2006a].

A meta-analysis of four phase III clinical trials of ibandronate in 8710 postmenopausal women with at least 2 years' follow-up showed that an annual cumulative exposure (ACE) ≥10.8 mg was associated with significant reductions in key nonvertebral fractures, all nonvertebral fractures, and all clinical fractures compared with placebo, at respective hazard ratios of 0.656, 0.701, and 0.712 [Harris et al. 2008]. The time to fracture was also significantly longer with an ACE ≥10.8 mg versus placebo at 2 years [Harris et al. 2008]. Furthermore, a pooled analysis of eight randomized trials of ibandronate in 9753 postmenopausal women with osteoporosis with 1–3 years' follow-up indicated that an annual cumulative exposure of ≥10.8 mg was associated with a significant reduction in nonvertebral fracture risk compared with an ACE of ≤7.2 mg and an ACE of 5.5 mg, at respective hazard ratios of 0.635 and 0.621 [Cranney, 2009]. There was also a significant dose–response effect seen with ACEs of 7.2–12 mg compared with an ACE of 5.5 mg, at hazard ratios of 0.746–0.573 [Cranney, 2009].

A phase III trial of intravenous zoledronic acid 5 mg once yearly in 7765 postmenopausal osteoporotic women showed that the incidence of vertebral fracture was reduced by 70% compared with placebo after 3 years of treatment, while the incidence of hip fracture was reduced by 41% [Black et al. 2007]. Analysis of 2127 patients who had undergone repair of a hip fracture randomized to zoledronic acid or placebo and followed for 1.9 years indicated that zoledronic acid reduced the risk of nonvertebral fracture, at a hazard ratio of 0.73 [Lyles et al. 2007]. In addition, treatment with zoledronic acid was associated with improved survival; with the number of deaths during follow-up for patients treated with zoledronic acid was 9.6% and 13.3% for placebo patients, giving a hazard ratio of mortality with zoledronic acid of 0.72 [Lyles et al. 2007]. Zoledronic acid also significantly improved BMD compared with placebo after 3 years, at between-group differences of 6.02%, 6.71%, and 5.06% in total hip, lumbar spine, and femoral neck BMD, and improved indices of bone strength [Black et al. 2007]. It has also been shown that zoledronic acid decreases serum CTX by 49–52%, compared with 8% with placebo [Woodis, 2008].

The most common adverse effect with oral bisphosphonate treatment is mild gastrointestinal disturbances, which have been reduced by once-weekly formulations of alendronate and risedronate. Intravenous agents may induce a transient acute phase reaction, involving fever, and bone and muscle pain that improves or disappears with subsequent treatment [Kanis et al. 2008].

A potential side effect associated with bisphosphonates, in the treatment of osteoporosis, Paget's disease and metastatic bone disease, is osteonecrosis of the jaw (ONJ). The incidence of ONJ in the general population is unknown; this rare condition also may occur in patients not receiving bisphosphonates. Case reports have discussed ONJ development in patients with multiple myeloma or metastatic breast cancer receiving bisphosphonates as palliation for bone metastases. These patients are also receiving chemotherapeutic agents that might impair the immune system and affect angiogenesis. The incidence or prevalence of ONJ in patients taking bisphosphonates for osteoporosis seems to be very rare (1/100,000 patient-years). No causative relationship has been unequivocally demonstrated between ONJ and bisphosphonate therapy. A majority of ONJ occurs after tooth extraction. Furthermore, the underlying risk of developing ONJ may be increased in osteoporotic patients by comorbid diseases. Treatment for ONJ is generally conservative [Rizzoli et al. 2008b].

Bisphosphonates are strong antiresorptives that accumulate in bone. Preclinical studies using doses five times higher than the dose used in humans have shown that the marked suppression of bone turnover is associated with microcracks [Mashiba et al. 2000], raising issues about the optimal duration of treatment.

Calcitonin

Calcitonin is a naturally occurring hormone that, when given at pharmacologic doses, inhibits osteoclast activity and, hence, reduces bone resorption. As salmon calcitonin is 40–50 times more potent than human calcitonin, this has been used in the majority of clinical trials. It is, however, only registered for use in some countries. Traditionally, it has been given by subcutaneous or intramuscular injection, which is associated with a number of adverse effects, including gastrointestinal effects, and facial flushing. Nasal administration is more convenient and is associated with fewer adverse effects, but it is expensive [Brown & Josse, 2002; Reginster & Franchimont, 1985; Reginster et al. 1995]. Calcitonin may reduce the risk of vertebral fractures (Figure 4.18), but the degree of benefit is unclear and there appears to be no effect on nonvertebral fractures [Chesnut et al. 2000]. Because of an apparent analgesic effect, calcitonin is sometimes considered for patients with painful vertebral fractures.

Denosumab

The human monoclonal antibody denosumab binds to receptor activator of nuclear factor kappa B ligand (RANKL) with high affinity and specificity and inhibits its action [McClung et al. 2006]. A phase II randomized trial of 412 postmenopausal women with low BMD randomized to denosumab 6, 14, or 30 mg every 3 months, denosumab 14, 60, 100, or 210 mg every 6 months, open-label oral alendronate 70 mg once weekly, or placebo for 12 months showed that denosumab increased BMD at the lumbar spine by 3.0–6.7%, compared with 4.6% with alendronate and −0.8% with placebo [McClung et al. 2006]. Total hip increases were 1.9–3.6%, 2.1%, and −0.6%, respectively, while those at the distal third of the radius were 0.4–1.3%, −0.5%, and −2.0%, respectively [McClung et al. 2006]. CTX significantly decreased with denosumab compared with placebo as early as 3 days after administration, at reductions of 88% versus 6% [McClung et al. 2006]. BSAP levels also decreased significantly with denosumab [McClung et al. 2006]. In a 36-month extension of the trial involving 262 patients from the original cohort, denosumab continued at 6-monthly intervals was associated with increases in BMD of 9.4–11.8% over baseline at the lumbar spine, and 4.0–6.1% over baseline for the total hip [Miller et al. 2008]. In addition, one turnover markers were also consistently suppressed [Miller et al. 2008]. While discontinuing denosumab for 12 months led to decreases in BMD, resumption of treatment for 12 months was linked to increases in lumbar spine BMD of 9.0% over baseline and total hip BMD of 3.9% over baseline [Miller et al. 2008]. A separate 2-year, phase III investigation in 332 postmenopausal women indicated that denosumab significantly improves hip structural parameters over placebo and significantly reduces serum CTX, tartrate-resistant acid phosphatase 5b, and PINP [Bone et al. 2008]. All three investigations revealed that there were no significant differences in the number of adverse events between denosumab and placebo, with the most common adverse events in both treatment groups being arthralgia, nasopharyngitis, and back pain [Miller et al. 2008; Bone et al. 2008].

The results of the Fracture REduction Evaluation of Denosumab in Osteoporosis every 6 Months (FREEDOM) phase III trial, for which the primary outcome was the effect of denosumab on the risk of new vertebral fractures, have recently been published. In this study 60 mg of denosumab every 6 months reduced, after 3 years, the risk of new vertebral fractures by 68%, hip fracture risk by 40% and nonvertebral fracture risk by 20%. The overall tolerance profile appears to be satisfactory. Full-length publication of these results should be available in the coming months [Cummings et al. 2009].

Bone-forming agents

Peptides of the parathyroid hormone family

Peptides of the parathyroid hormone (PTH) family (Figure 4.19) have been investigated in the management of osteoporosis for more than 30 years [Reginster et al. 1997; Neuprez & Reginster, 2008]. A continuous endogenous production or exogenous administration of PTH, as is the case in primary or secondary hyperparathyroidism, can lead to deleterious consequences for the skeleton, particularly for cortical bone. However, intermittent administration of PTH (eg, through daily subcutaneous injections) results in an increase in the number and activity of osteoblasts, leading to an increase in bone mass (Figure 4.20) and an improvement in skeletal architecture at both the trabecular and cortical skeleton. This treatment also increases cortical bone width.

The full length (1–84) PTH molecule and the 1–34 N-terminal fragment are currently used for the management of osteoporosis. Based on their respective molecular weights, an equivalent dose of the 1–34 fragment, relative to the 1–84 molecule, is 40% (eg, 20 and 40 µg of 1–34 PTH is equivalent to 50 and 100 µg of 1–84 PTH, respectively).

In order to assess the effects of the 1–34 N-terminal fragment of PTH on fractures (Figures 4.21–4.22), 1637 postmenopausal women with prior spine fractures were randomly assigned to receive 20 or 40 µg of 1–34 PTH or placebo, subcutaneously self-administered daily. Spine radiographs were obtained at baseline and at the end of the study (median duration of observation, 21 months), and serial measurements of bone mass were performed by dual-X-ray absorptiometry. New spine fractures occurred in 14% of the women in the placebo group and in 5% and 4% of the women in the 20- and 40-µg dose groups, respectively. The relative risk of fracture, as compared with the placebo group, was 0.35 and 0.31 (95% CI 0.22–0.55 and 0.19–0.50), respectively. New non-spine fractures occurred in 6% of the women in the placebo group and 3% of those in each PTH group (Relative risk [RR] 0.47 and 0.46, 95% CI 0.25–0.88 and 0.25–0.86, respectively). PTH had only minor side-effects (occasional nausea and headache) [Neer et al. 2001].

The antifracture efficacy of PTH on spine fracture was not modulated by the age of the subjects (<65 years of age, 65–75 years of age or >75 years of age), prevalent spinal bone mineral density (BMD) values (T-score less than −2.5 or greater than −2.5) or number of prevalent fractures (one or two or more fractures) [Marcus et al. 2003].

At the end of this trial, patients were followed for an additional 18-month period without PTH, during which they were allowed to use any antiosteoporotic medication considered appropriate by their care-giver. Although the proportion of patients having received an inhibitor of bone resorption was slightly higher in patients previously in the placebo group than in the patients having received PTH 20 µg/day, the reduction of spine fractures observed in this particular group during the initial trial was confirmed during this 18-month period (RR 0.59; 95% CI 0.42–0.85) [Lindsay et al. 2004]. A follow-up in 1262 women was conducted up to 30 months after discontinuation of treatment. The hazard ratio for combined teriparatide groups (20 and 40 µg) for the 50-month period after baseline was 0.57 (95% CI 0.40–0.82), suggesting a sustained effect in reducing the risk of non-spine fragility fracture [Prince et al. 2005].

Teriparatide-mediated relative fracture risk reduction was shown to be independent of pretreatment bone turnover, demonstrating that this therapy offers clinical benefit to patients across a range of disease severity [Delmas et al. 2006b].

Full-length recombinant human PTH (1–84) has also been investigated in the management of postmenopausal osteoporosis. It has been postulated that the C-terminal region of PTH, which teriparatide lacks, also has biological functions in the bone that are mediated by a novel receptor specific for this region of the hormone. Teriparatide, for instance, has been associated with osteosarcoma in rats treated with massive doses during most of their lifespan, possibly related to its antiapoptotic effects in bone cells and decrease in production of C-terminal PTH fragments. In contrast, researchers suggest that PTH (1–84) is likely not to have such an effect due to the pro-apoptotic effects of C-terminal PTH fragments that maintain normal bone cell turnover [Jilka et al. 1999; Greenspan et al. 2007]. In a phase II study, women self-administered PTH (50, 75 or 100 μg) or placebo by daily subcutaneous injection for 12 months. The 100 μg dose increased BMD significantly at 3 months and 12 months (+7.8%). Bone area also significantly increased (+2.0%). A non-significant decrease (−0.9%) in total hip BMD occurred during the first 6 months with the 100-μg dose, but this trend reversed (+1.6%) during the second 6 months. Bone turnover markers increased during the first half of the study and were maintained at elevated levels during the second 6 months. Dose-related incidences of transient hypercalcemia occurred, but only one patient (in the 100 μg group) was withdrawn because of repeated hypercalcemia [Greenspan et al. 2007; Shrader & Raggucci, 2005]. Results from the pivotal phase III studies have not yet been published as full papers. Evidence from the TOP (treatment of osteoporosis with parathyroid hormone) study, including women with low BMD (with or without previous fracture), suggests that PTH (1–84) reduced the incidence of vertebral fractures in all patients and prevented the incidence of a first vertebral fracture in women with postmenopausal osteoporosis [Greenspan et al. 2007]. Reduction of nonvertebral or hip fractures does not clearly appear from the currently available data [Shrader & Raggucci, 2005; Hodsman et al. 2003; 2005].

Strontium ranelate

Strontium ranelate is a new treatment of postmenopausal osteoporosis that reduces the risk of vertebral and hip fractures. It is the first antiosteoporotic agent that appears to simultaneously increase bone formation (Figure 4.23) and decrease bone resorption, thus uncoupling the bone remodeling process [Reginster et al. 2007]. Specifically, the dual mode of action of strontium ranelate (Figure 4.24) is due to direct effects on both osteoblasts and osteoclasts, as reflectected by the changes in bone markers in clinical trials [Meunier et al. 2004]. Several studies in various models have demonstrated that strontium ranelate increases osteoblast replication, differentiation, and activity, [Canalis et al. 1996] while in parallel, it downregulates osteoclast differentiation and activity [Baron & Tsouderos, 2002; Takahashi et al. 2003; Hurtel Lemaire et al. 2009]. A recent study has shown that strontium ranelate increases the expression of the bone-specific alkaline phosphatase (osteoblast differentiation) and the number of the bone nodules (osteoblast activity) of murine osteoblasts. In parallel, strontium ranelate decreases the tartrate resistant acid phosphatase activity (osteoclast differentiation) and the capability of murine osteoclasts to resorb (osteoclast activity), probably by acting on the cytoskeleton of these cells [Bonnelye et al. 2008]. In addition to these direct effects on osteoblasts and osteoclasts, strontium ranelate also modulates the level of osteoprotegerin (OPG) and RANKL, two molecules strongly involved in the regulation of osteoclastogenesis by osteoblasts. Other studies have demonstrated the involvement of the calcium-sensing receptor in the effects of strontium ranelate on osteoblasts, osteoclasts, OPG/RANKL regulation [Hurtel Lemaire et al. 2009].

Strontium ranelate has been investigated in a large phase III program, initiated in 1996, which includes two extensive clinical trials for the treatment of osteoporosis [Meunier et al. 2004; Reginster et al. 2005; 2009]. The SOTI (Spinal Osteoporosis Therapeutic Intervention) study was aimed at assessing the effect of strontium ranelate on the risk of vertebral fractures [Meunier et al. 2004] (Figure 4.25). The TROPOS (Treatment Of Peripheral Osteoporosis) trial aimed to evaluate the effect of strontium ranelate on peripheral (nonspinal) fractures [Reginster et al. 2005] (Figure 4.26).

Both studies were multinational, randomized, double-blind, and placebo-controlled, with two parallel groups (strontium ranelate 2 g/day vs. placebo) [Meunier et al. 2004; Reginster et al. 2005]. The study duration was 5 years, with main statistical analysis planned after 3 years of follow-up. 1649 patients were included in SOTI (mean age 70 years), and 5091 patients were included in TROPOS (mean age 77 years) [Reginster et al. 2002].

The primary analysis of SOTI [Meunier et al. 2004] (intention to treat [ITT], n=1442), evaluating the effect of strontium ranelate 2 g/day on vertebral fracture rates, revealed a 41% reduction in relative risk of experiencing a new vertebral fracture (semiquantitative assessment) with strontium ranelate throughout the 3-year study compared with placebo (139 patients with vertebral fracture vs. 222, respectively [RR 0.59; 95% CI: 0.48, 0.73; $p<0.001$]). The RR of experiencing a new vertebral fracture was significantly reduced in the strontium ranelate group as compared with the placebo group for the first year. Over the first 12 months, RR reduction was 49% (RR 0.51; 95% CI: 0.36, 0.74, respectively; Cox model $p<0.001$).

The primary analysis of TROPOS (ITT, n=4932), evaluating the effect of strontium ranelate 2 g/day on nonvertebral fracture, showed a 16% RR reduction in all nonvertebral fractures over a 3-year follow-up period (RR 0.84; 95% CI: 0.702, 0.995; $p=0.04$) [Reginster et al. 2005]. Strontium ranelate treatment was associated with a 19% reduction in risk of major nonvertebral osteoporotic fractures (RR 0.81; 95% CI: 0.66, 0.98; $p=0.031$). In the high-risk fracture subgroup (n=1977; women; mean age ≥74 years; femoral-neck BMD T-score of less than or equal to −2.4 according to National Health and Nutrition Examination Survey [NHANES] normative value), treatment was associated with a 36% reduction in risk of hip fracture (RR 0.64; 95% CI: 0.412, 0.997; $p=0.046$).

Of the 5091 patients, 2714 (53%) completed the study up to 5 years [Reginster et al. 2008a]. The risk of nonvertebral fracture was reduced by 15% in the strontium ranelate group compared with the placebo group (RR 0.85; 95% CI: 0.73, 0.99). The risk of hip fracture was decreased by 43% (RR 0.57; 95% CI: 0.33, 0.97), and the risk of vertebral fracture was decreased by 24% (RR 0.76; 95% CI: 0.65, 0.88) in the strontium ranelate group. After 5 years, the safety profile of strontium ranelate remained unchanged compared with the 3-year findings [Reginster et al. 2008a].

In order to assess the efficacy of strontium ranelate according to the main determinants of vertebral fracture risk (age, baseline BMD, prevalent fractures, family history of osteoporosis, baseline BMI, and addiction to smoking), data from SOTI and TROPOS (n=5082) were pooled (strontium ranelate 2 g/day group [n=2536]; placebo group [n=2546]; average age 74 years; 3-year follow up) [Roux et al. 2006]. Strontium ranelate decreased the risk of both vertebral (RR 0.60; 95% CI: 0.53, 0.69; $p<0.001$) and nonvertebral (RR 0.85; 95% CI: 0.74, 0.99; $p=0.03$) fractures. The decrease in risk of vertebral fractures was 37% (P=0.003) in women aged <70 years, 42% ($p<0.001$) for those aged 70 to 80 years, and 32% ($p=0.013$) for those aged ≥80 years. The RR of vertebral fracture was 0.28 (95% CI: 0.07, 0.99) in osteopenic and 0.61 (95% CI: 0.53, 0.70) in osteoporotic women, and baseline BMD was not a determinant of efficacy.

This study showed that a 3-year treatment with strontium ranelate leads to antivertebral fracture efficacy in postmenopausal women independently of baseline osteoporotic risk factors [Roux et al. 2006].

To determine whether strontium ranelate also reduces fractures in elderly patients, an analysis based on preplanned pooling of data from the SOTI and TROPOS trials included 1488 women between 80 and 100 years of age followed for 3 years [Seeman et al. 2006]. In the ITT analysis, the risk of vertebral, nonvertebral, and clinical (symptomatic vertebral and nonvertebral) fractures was reduced within 1 year by 59% ($p=0.002$), 41% ($p=0.027$), and 37% ($p=0.012$), respectively. At the end of 3 years, vertebral, nonvertebral, and clinical fracture risks were reduced by 32% ($p=0.013$), 31% ($p=0.011$), and 22% ($p=0.040$), respectively. The medication was well tolerated, and the safety profile was similar to that in younger patients.

Strontium ranelate was studied in 1431 postmenopausal women with osteopenia [Seeman et al. 2008]. In women with lumbar spine osteopenia, strontium ranelate decreased the risk of vertebral fracture by 41% (RR 0.59; 95% CI: 0.43, 0.82; p=0.002), by 59% in women with no prevalent fractures (RR 0.41; 95% CI: 0.17, 0.99; p=0.039), and by 38% in women with prevalent fractures (RR 0.62; 95% CI: 0.44, 0.88; p=0.008). In women with osteopenia both at the lumbar spine and the femoral neck, strontium ranelate reduced the risk of fracture by 52% (RR 0.48; 95% CI: 0.24, 0.96; p=0.034).

After 3 years of strontium ranelate 2 g/day, each percentage point increase in femoral neck and total proximal femur BMD was associated with a 3% (95% adjusted CI: 1, 5) and 2% (CI: 1, 4) reduction in risk of new vertebral fracture, respectively. The 3-year changes in femoral neck and total proximal femur BMD explained 76% and 74% of the reduction in vertebral fractures observed during the treatment, respectively [Bruyère et al. 2007].

In the SOTI and TROPOS trials, the incidence of adverse events, serious adverse events, and withdrawals due to adverse events was similar in the strontium ranelate and placebo groups [Shea et al. 2004; European Medicines Agency, 2007]. During the first 3 months of treatment, nausea, diarrhea, headache, dermatitis, and eczema were more frequently associated with strontium ranelate compared to placebo; but, thereafter, there was no difference in incidence between strontium ranelate and placebo groups with respect to nausea and diarrhea.

In pooled data from the SOTI and TROPOS trials, there was an apparent increased risk of VTE in the strontium ranelate group (0.6% vs. 0.9% per year), although the annual incidence was similar in the strontium ranelate and placebo groups in the individual trials [Meunier, 2004; Reginster et al. 2005].

A recently published study used the UK General Practice Research Database to assess the risk of several recently reported adverse events linked to the use of strontium ranelate for osteoporosis in postmenopausal women [Grosso, 2008]. Age-adjusted rate ratios for VTE, gastrointestinal disturbance, minor skin complaint and memory loss were 1.1 (95% CI: 0.2, 5.0), 3.0 (95% CI: 2.3, 3.8), 2.0 (95% CI: 1.3, 3.1), and 1.8 (95% CI: 0.2, 14.1), respectively. No cases of osteonecrosis of the jaw, Stevens–Johnson syndrome or drug rash with eosinophilia and systemic symptoms were found.

Long-term management of postmenopausal osteoporosis

There have been few studies examining the long-term pharmacological management of postmenopausal osteoporosis.

The Fracture Intervention Trial Long-term Extension (FLEX) trial showed that, among postmenopausal women who had received alendronate for 5 years, continuing alendronate 5 or 10 mg/day for a further 5 years had no impact on the cumulative vertebral fracture risk compared with switching to placebo for 5 years, at a relative risk of 1.00 [Black et al. 2006]. While there was a significantly lower risk of clinical vertebral fracture with continuing alendronate for a further 5 years compared with switching to placebo, at a relative risk of 0.45, there was no reduction in the risk of morphometric vertebral fractures [Black et al. 2006]. Switching to placebo was associated with declines in BMD at the total hip and spine and increases in serum markers of born turnover [Black et al. 2006]. However, levels did not reach pretreatment levels observed 10 years earlier [Black et al. 2006].

So far, strontium ranelate is the only treatment having demonstrated an efficacy over 5 years against vertebral, nonvertebral and hip fractures in a phase III, double-blind, placebo-controlled, preplanned study. In addition, the very long-term efficacy of strontium ranelate has been investigated in an extension of the SOTI and TROPOS studies, in which a total of 879 patients were entered into a 3-year open-label extension to examine the impact of administration over 8 years [Reginster et al. 2008]. The cumulative incidence of vertebral fractures over the extension was 13.7%, compared with 11.5% in the first 3 years of the combined original trials, while the cumulative incidence of nonvertebral fractures was 12.0%, compared with 9.6% in the first 3 years of the study [Reginster et al. 2008a]. Despite an increased fracture risk with ageing, there was no significant difference in vertebral and nonvertebral fracture risk between the original trial periods and the open-label extensions illustrating the maintenance of antifracture efficacy of this agent [Reginster et al. 2008a]. There were no additional safety concerns [Reginster et al. 2008a].

Guidelines for the treatment of women with postmenopausal osteoporosis

Figure 4.1. The decision of how to treat postmenopausal osteoporosis should be based on an assessment of fracture risk, and the efficacy and adverse effects of the drugs likely to be prescribed. In general, women who meet the criteria listed in this figure are probable candidates for treatment. Algorithms have been developed to establish the 10-year probability of all low trauma fractures according to age, history of fractures, bone mass, and level of bone resorption, which can be used when assessing treatment options. BMD, bone mineral density. Adapted with permission from the American Association of Clinical Endocrinologists. Medical guidelines for clinical practice for the prevention and treatment of postmenopausal osteoporosis: 2001 edition, with selected updates for 2003. Endocr Pract 2003; 9:544–64.

Which women should be treated with pharmacological therapy for osteoporosis?	Examples
Women with postmenopausal osteoporosis	Eg, as shown either by a low BMD or the presence of osteoporotic fractures
Women with borderline BMD measurements	If additional risk factors are present
Women in whom nonpharmacological preventative measures have been ineffective	Eg, if bone loss continues, or low-trauma fractures occur

Nonpharmacologic approaches to the prevention of postmenopausal osteoporosis and osteoporotic fractures

Figure 4.2. There are a number of nonpharmacologic approaches for the prevention of postmenopausal osteoporosis and osteoporotic fractures, which are outlined in the figure below. The recommended calcium intake for postmenopausal women is 1000–1500 mg/day, and vitamin D up to 800 IU/day. Exercise programs should be encouraged, but not those that could do harm, such as back flexion exercises in patients with vertebral osteoporosis. In order to minimize falls, the home environment should be checked to remove any obstacles that could cause falls, and handrails should be added where necessary.

Advise postmenopausal patients of the risk factors for osteoporosis

- Lifestyle changes
- Advise an adequate intake of dietary calcium
- Advise regular, suitable weight-bearing, and muscle-strengthening exercise
- Advise, and help patients who smoke to stop
- Advise patients to drink alcohol at safe levels

Minimize risk of falls

- Avoid drugs with sedative effects, or reduce dosage if possible
- Identify, and treat sensory deficits that can contribute to falls
- Identify, and treat neurologic and rheumatologic conditions that can contribute to falls
- Instigate gait and balance training if necessary
- In elderly women, consider occupational therapy to provide household items, such as anchor rugs, non-skid mats, and to advise on home modifications, such as improved lighting, and handrails

Recommend hip protectors in those prone to falls

Effects of exercising on bone density

Figure 4.3. (a) The effects of exercise on bone density were studied, and found to depend on the site of maximal change in the stress–strain relationship. Greater changes in bone mineral density (BMD) were generally seen with strength exercise regimens than endurance exercise regimens (which do not increase the stress–strain relationship), especially in the trochanteric and intertrochanteric areas. **(b)** In women with postmenopausal osteoporosis who performed supervised aerobic, weight-bearing, and weight-lifting exercises three times per week it was found that they had increased femoral neck, trochanteric, and lumbar spine BMD compared with women who did not exercise. These effects were enhanced in women who were taking hormone replacement therapy as well as exercising. Adapted from Going S, Lohman T, Houtkooper L et al. Effects of exercise on bone mineral density in calcium-replete postmenopausal women with and without hormone replacement therapy. Osteoporos Int 2003; 14:637–43.

(a)

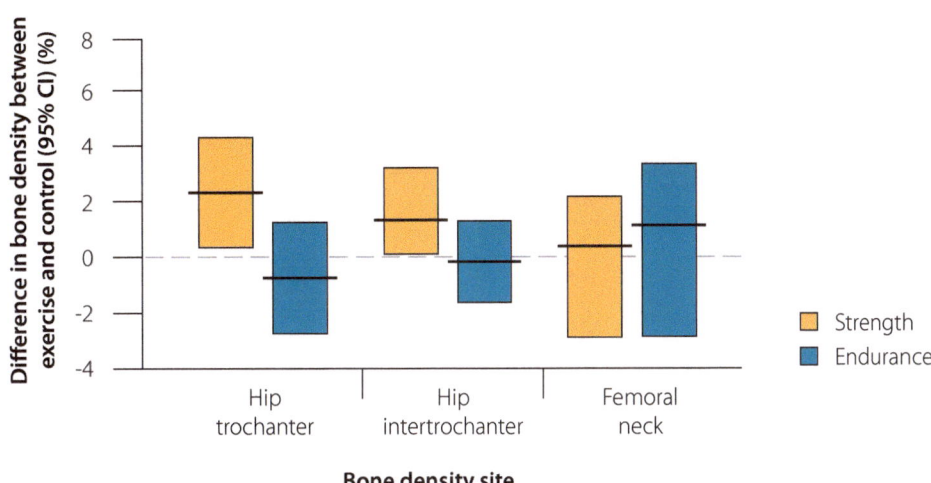

(b)

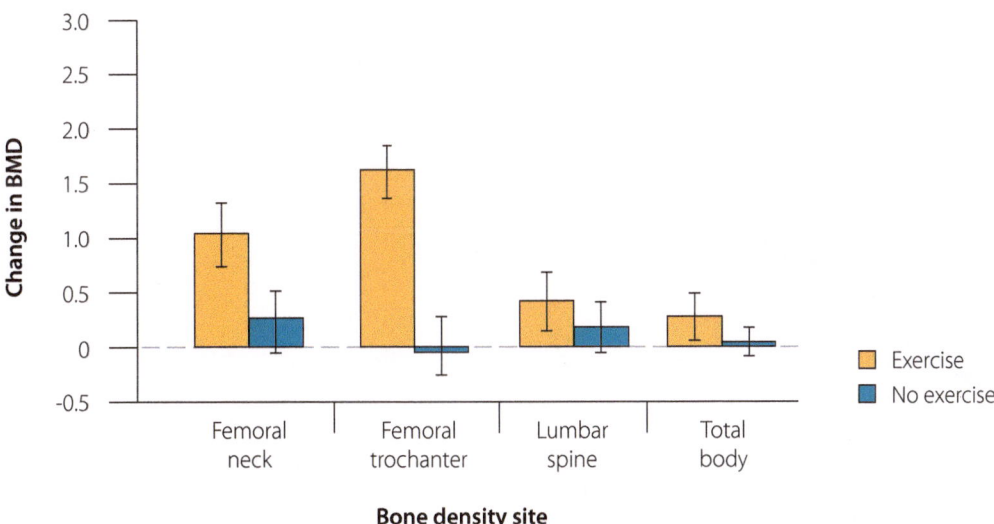

Effects of calcium plus vitamin D on fractures in elderly institutionalized women

Figure 4.4. In a study of elderly women in institutional care who had inadequate intake of both calcium and vitamin D (mean age 84 years), calcium and vitamin D supplementation (tricalcium phosphate 1.2 g plus cholecalciferol 800 IU) was found to not only prevent bone loss, but also to reduce hip fractures by 43% **(a)**, and nonvertebral fractures by 32% **(b)** compared with placebo. Data from Chapuy MC, Arlot ME, Duboeuf F et al. Vitamin D3 and calcium to prevent hip fractures in the elderly women. N Engl J Med 1992; 327:1637–42.

(a)

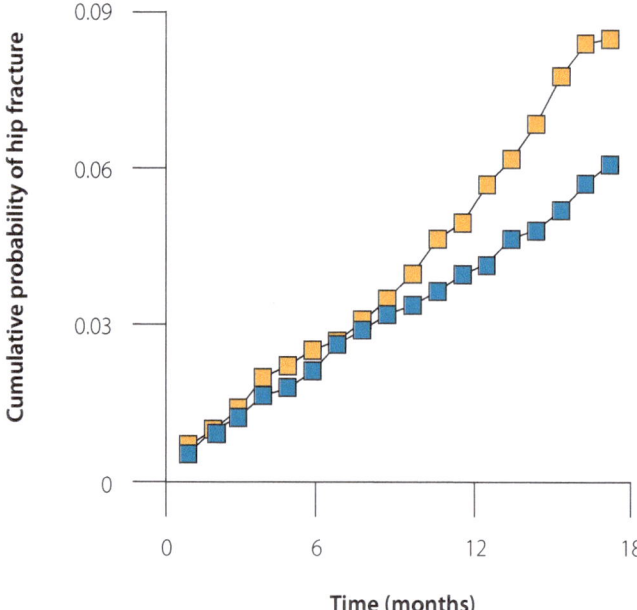

(b)

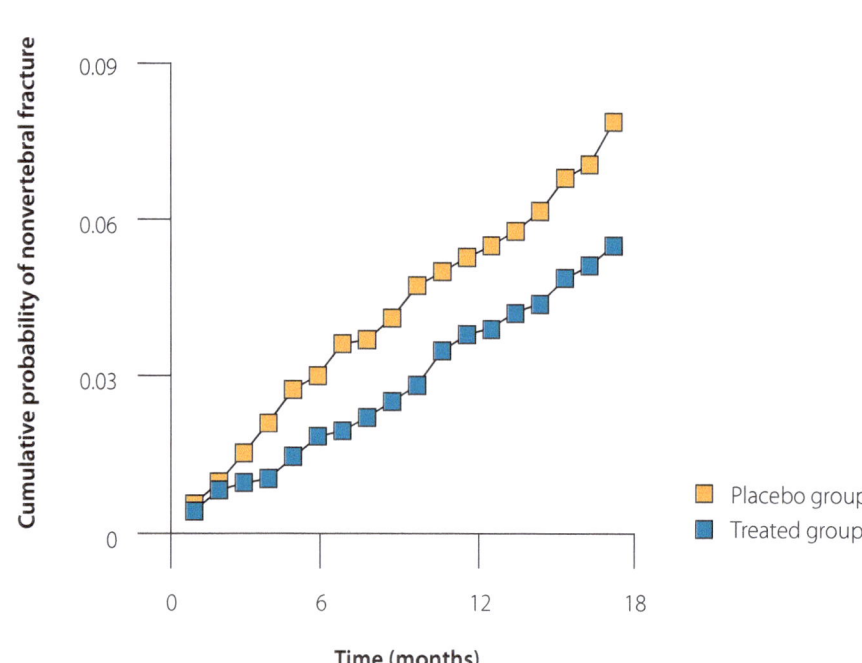

The hip protector

Figure 4.5. In the elderly, it is more common to fall sideways onto the hip rather than forwards onto hands or knees as with younger people. The direct impact of a sideways fall is on the greater trochanter of the proximal femur, which can result in hip fracture. There has, therefore, been interest in finding a device that can protect the hips and prevent fracture, to allow the force and energy of a fall to be attenuated and shunted away from the greater trochanter. One such device is the external hip protector, which has been found to reduce the risk of hip fracture by up to 80% in those at increased risk for hip fracture, when it is being worn at the time of the fall. There is, however, poor compliance with wearing hip protectors owing to discomfort and impracticality, and they are usually not worn at night. Compliance difficulties may be reduced through the use of education programs.

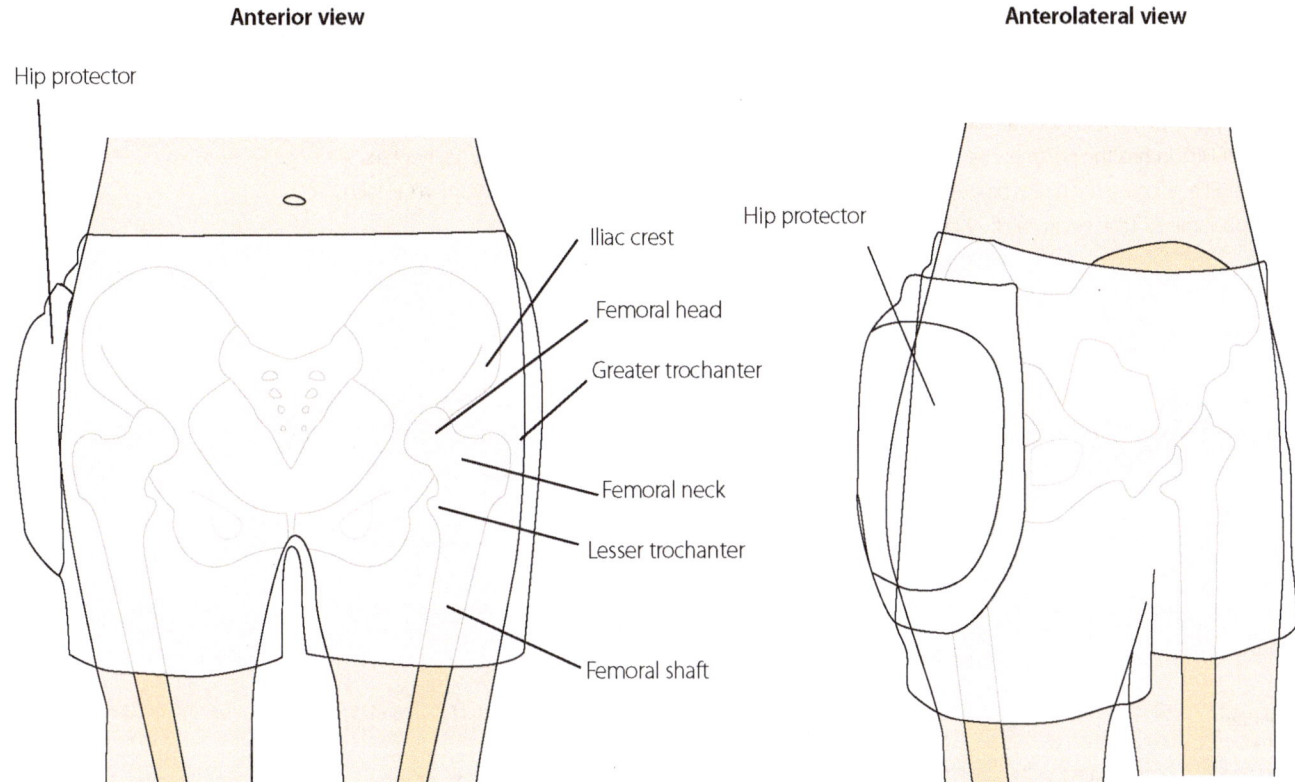

97

Kaplan-Meier estimates of cumulative hazards for fracture with hormone replacement therapy

Figure 4.6. The Women's Health Initiative (WHI) study is the largest clinical trial of hormone replacement therapy (HRT) ever conducted in postmenopausal women aged 50–79 years with an intact uterus at baseline [Cauley, 2003]. In the HRT arm of the study, some 16,600 postmenopausal women were randomly allocated to receive placebo or HRT (conjugated equine estrogen 0.625 mg/day plus medroxyprogesterone acetate 2.5 mg/day). The multiple outcomes evaluated in this study included heart disease, stroke, venous thromboembolism, and breast, uterine, and colon cancer, as well as fractures. The principal results of the study showed that 44 (0.1%) in the HRT group experienced hip fractures **(a)**, compared with 62 (0.15%) in the placebo group; 41 (0.09%) versus 60 (0.15%) experienced clinical vertebral fractures **(b)**; and 650 (1.47%) versus 780 (1.91%) experienced other types of fractures, respectively. The risk for all fractures is shown in **(c)**. The rates of observed hip and clinical vertebral fractures were reduced by 34% in the HRT group and the risk of all other fractures was reduced by 24% compared with placebo. This reduction was nominally significant for all fractures. With regard to absolute risk, 10,000 women receiving HRT might experience five fewer hip fractures over 1 year compared with placebo [Rossouw, 2002]. In a further analysis of the WHI results, 733 (8.6%) in the HRT group, and 896 (11.1%) in the placebo group experienced a fracture. After 3 years of treatment, total hip BMD was increased by 3.7% in the HRT group compared with 0.14% in the placebo group. The results from WHI have shown that the overall health risks outweigh the benefits of the use of HRT in healthy postmenopausal women. Reproduced with permission from Cauley JA, Robbins J, Chen Z et al. Effects of estrogen plus progestin on risk of fracture and bone mineral density. The Women's Health Initiative Randomized Trial. JAMA 2003; 290:1729–38.

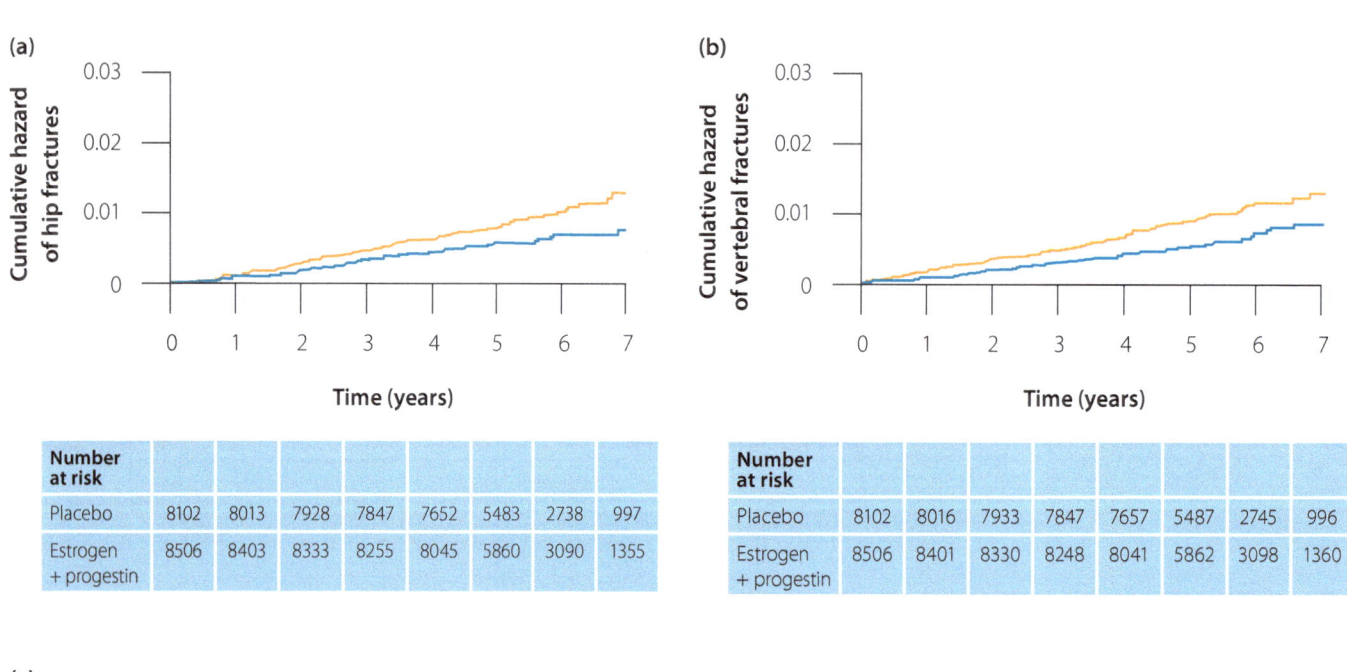

(a)

Number at risk								
Placebo	8102	8013	7928	7847	7652	5483	2738	997
Estrogen + progestin	8506	8403	8333	8255	8045	5860	3090	1355

(b)

Number at risk								
Placebo	8102	8016	7933	7847	7657	5487	2745	996
Estrogen + progestin	8506	8401	8330	8248	8041	5862	3098	1360

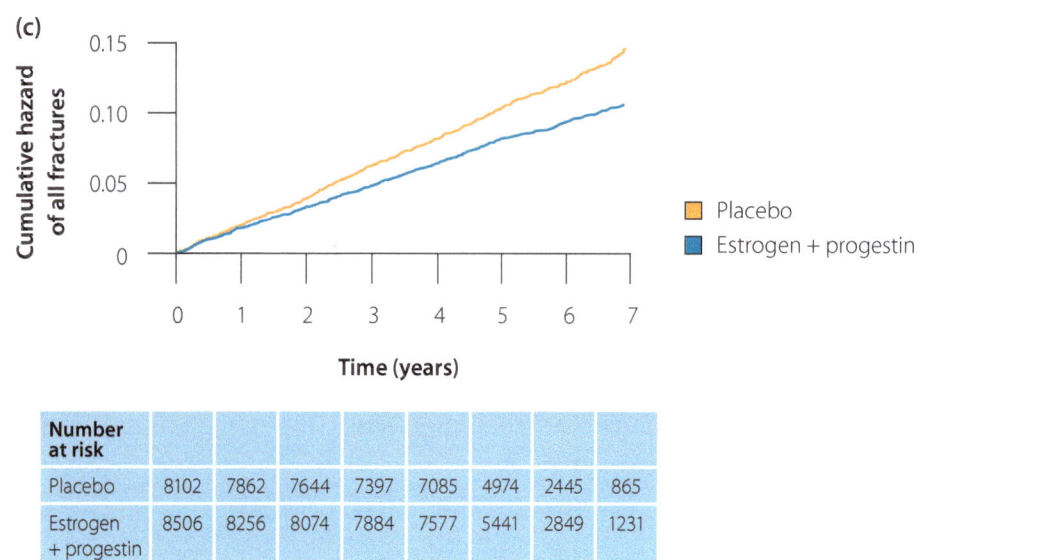

(c)

■ Placebo
■ Estrogen + progestin

Number at risk								
Placebo	8102	7862	7644	7397	7085	4974	2445	865
Estrogen + progestin	8506	8256	8074	7884	7577	5441	2849	1231

Mode of action of selective estrogen receptor modulators

Figure 4.7. The mode of action of selective estrogen receptor modulators (SERMs), such as raloxifene, is complex. All of the SERMs will bind to the estrogen receptor, but each compound has a slightly different shape. The binding of estrogen, antiestrogen, or SERMS to the receptor causes the receptor to undergo a conformational change that permits its spontaneous dimerization, and consequently enables it to interact with estrogen response elements (EREs), which are located within target genes. The different conformational structures of the estrogen-receptor–ligand complexes lead to binding of various coregulator proteins. For example, some estrogen-receptor–SERM complexes favor coactivator recruitment, which can increase agonist activity, while other SERMs may facilitate the interaction of the estrogen receptor with currently unknown coactivators with which estrogens, or antiestrogens, would not normally couple. Estrogen has been shown to facilitate the interaction of the estrogen receptor with coactivators, while the antagonist-activated estrogen receptor interacts preferentially with corepressors. This model implies that SERM activity will be influenced by the relative levels of expression of the coregulator proteins (corepressors and coactivator), which are expressed in different target cells. Reproduced with permission from Riggs BL, Hartmann LC. Selective estrogen-receptor modulators – mechanisms of action and application to clinical practice. N Engl J Med 2003; 348:618–9.

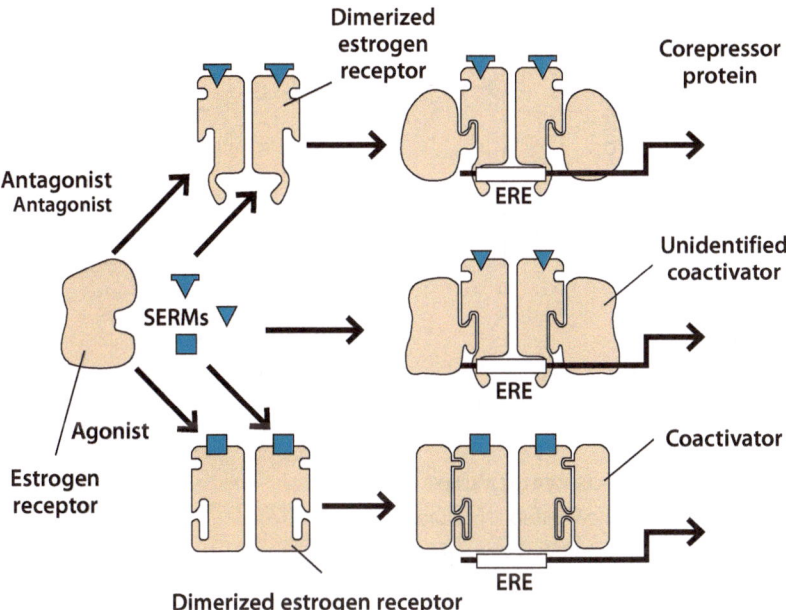

Structure of estradiol and raloxifene

Figure 4.8. Estradiol is a semisynthetic human estrogenic hormone used to treat menopausal symptoms, and to prevent osteoporosis in postmenopausal women. Raloxifene is a selective estrogen receptor modulator (SERM) that is used in the management of postmenopausal osteoporosis. There is a structural similarity between these two compounds that accounts for the estrogen-like effect of raloxifene on bone.

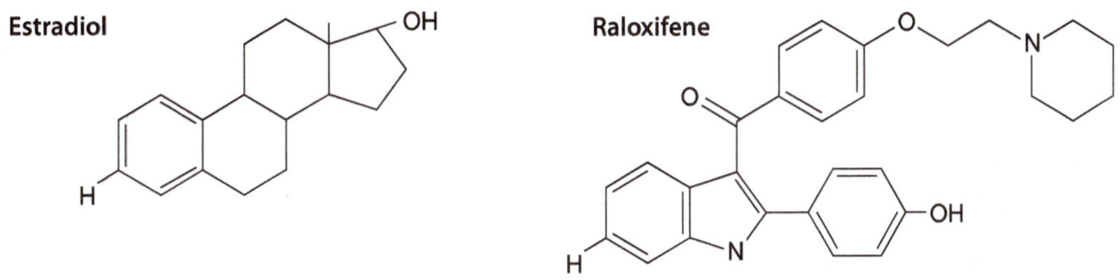

Estradiol

Raloxifene

Effects of raloxifene on lumbar spine and femoral neck bone mineral density

Figure 4.9. The effects of raloxifene on bone mineral density (BMD) at the lumbar spine **(a)** and femoral neck **(b)** are shown. The Multiple Outcomes of Raloxifene Evaluation (MORE) trial included postmenopausal women with known osteoporosis (low BMD, or prevalent vertebral fractures) who were randomly allocated to receive raloxifene (60 mg/day) or placebo. The results showed that there was a 2–3% increase in spine and hip BMD after 2 and 3 years of treatment compared with placebo. Adapted from Ettinger B, Black DM, Mitlak BH et al. Reduction of vertebral fracture risk in postmenopausal women with osteoporosis treated with raloxifene: results from a 3-year randomized clinical trial. JAMA 1999; 282:637–45.

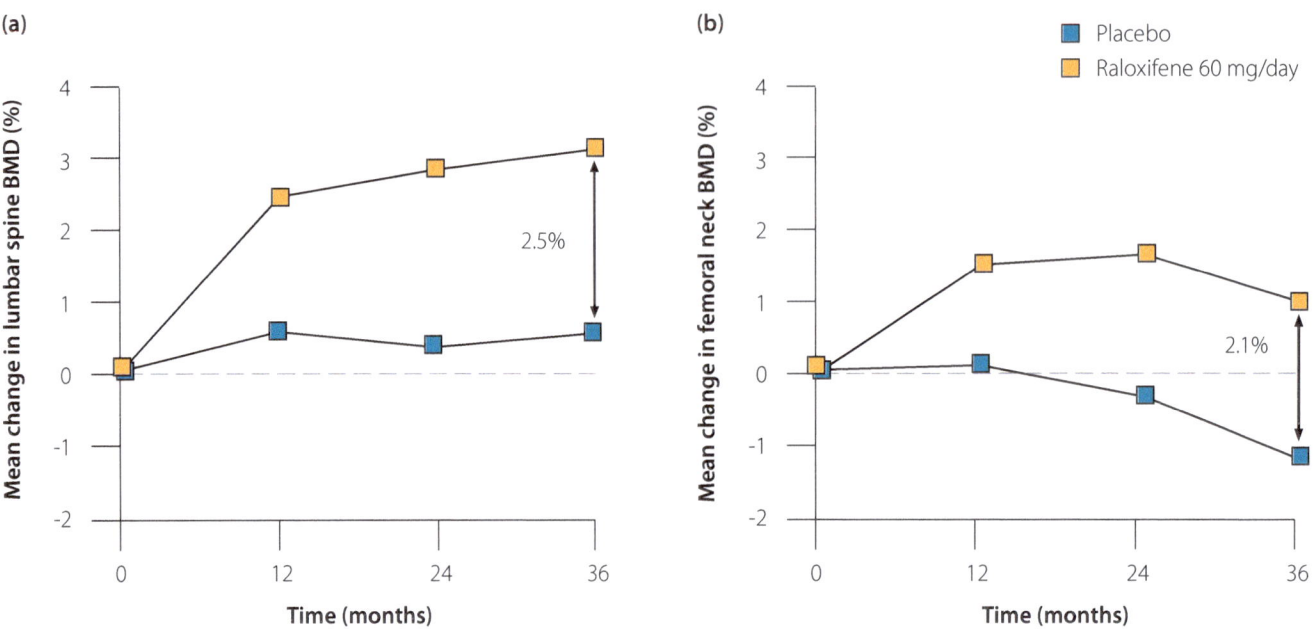

Effects of raloxifene on incidence of new vertebral fractures

Figure 4.10. The effects of raloxifene on risk of vertebral fracture are shown in subjects from the Multiple Outcomes of Raloxifene Evaluation (MORE) trial. After six months 503 (7.4%) had at least one new vertebral fracture, including 10.1% in the placebo-treated group and 6.6% of the raloxifene-treated group. The results showed that there was a decreased risk of new vertebral fractures from 30% to 50% with raloxifene treatment. This reduction was significant for women with and without vertebral fractures at baseline. RR, relative risk. Reproduced with permission from Ettinger B, Black DM, Mitlak BH et al. Reduction of vertebral fracture risk in postmenopausal women with osteoporosis treated with raloxifene: results from a 3-year randomized clinical trial. JAMA 1999; 282:637–45.

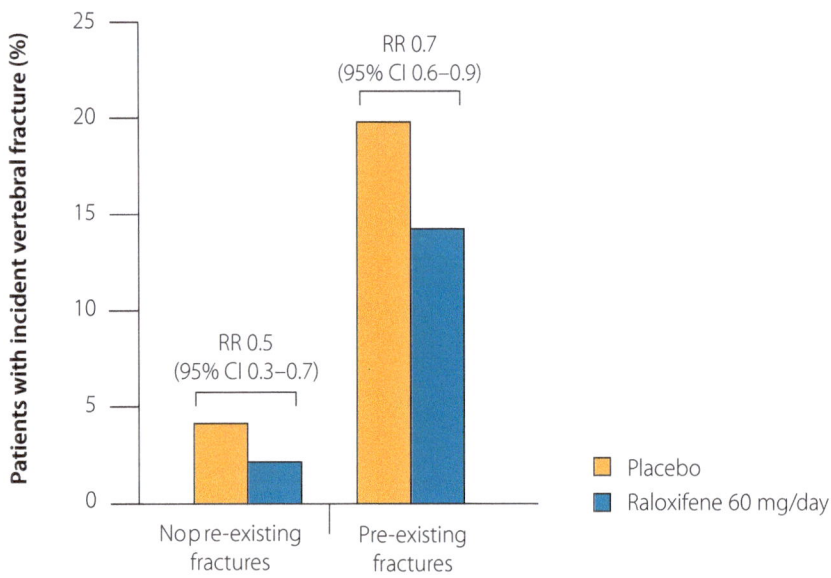

General structure of pyrophosphate and bisphosphonates

Figure 4.11. Bisphosphonates are analogs of pyrophosphate, which is characterized by two phosphoric acid groups bound to a central oxygen molecule. In pyrophosphate **(a)**, the phosphate–oxygen bonds are readily degraded by ubiquitous enzymes (pyrophosphatases), but in the bisphosphonates **(b)**, the phosphate–carbon bonds are essentially impervious to enzymatic degradation. The carbon of bisphosphonates has two side chains, R_1 and R_2, that can be substituted to determine the avidity of binding to bone, and the antiresorptive potency, respectively. The different side chains can also influence the adverse effects of these molecules. Adapted with permission from Watts NB. Bisphosphonate treatment for osteoporosis. In: The Osteoporotic Syndrome. Edited by LV Avioli. San Diego: Academic Press, 2000;121–32.

Action of bisphosphonates

Figure 4.12. Bisphosphonates owe their action to their ability to bind avidly to the surface of bone, especially where there is active remodeling of bone. The non-nitrogen-containing bisphosphonates (eg, etidronate) are metabolized to cytotoxic ATP-bisphosphonate analogs, whereas the nitrogen-containing bisphosphonates (eg, alendronate, risedronate, ibandronate, zoledronate) inhibit the mevalonic acid pathway, and the enzyme farnesyl pyrophosphatase, resulting in decreased osteoclastic activity, and a reduced rate of bone remodeling. There is a consequent reduction in bone formation and preservation of the bone architecture. ATP, adenosine triphosphate; BMD, bone mineral density. Adapted with permission from McClung MR. Bisphosphonates. Endcrinol Metab Clin North Am 2003; 32:253–71.

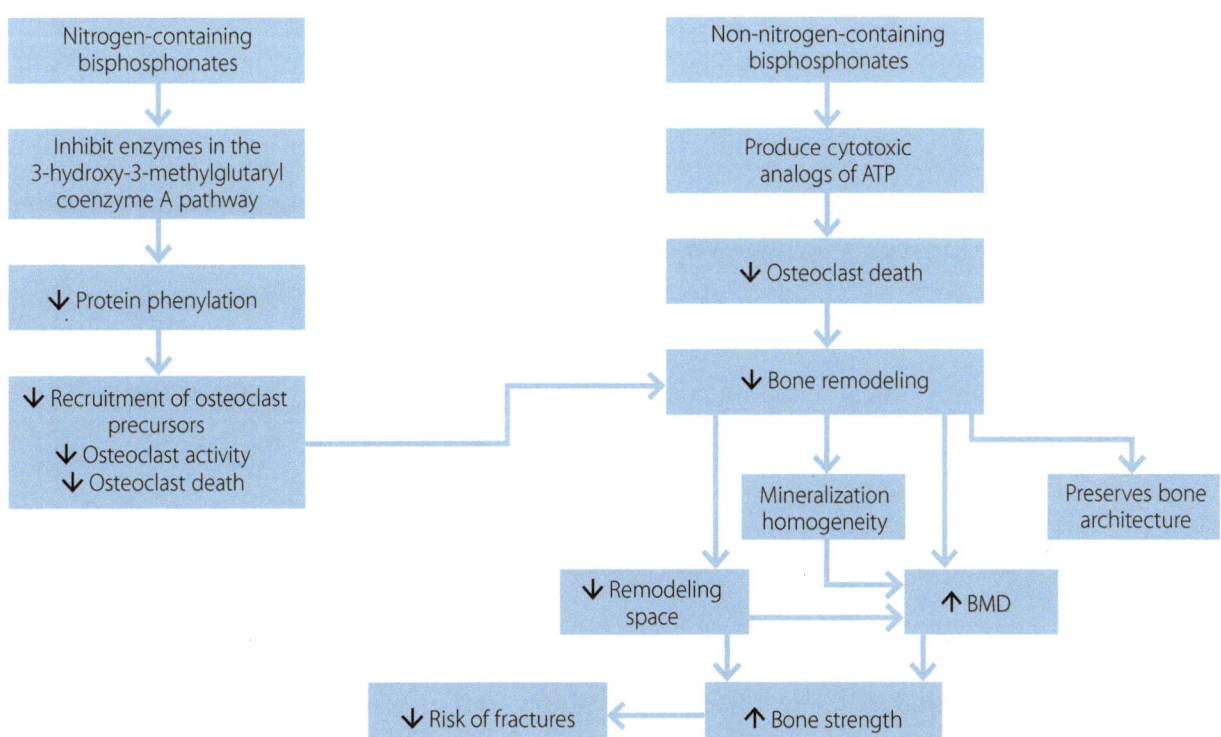

Effect of alendronate on risk of fractures

Figure 4.13. The Fracture Intervention Trial (FIT) also showed that alendronate was effective in reducing the risk of fractures. The percentage of patients having new fractures at three sites after 3 years of treatment with alendronate compared with placebo is shown. In the study, 8.0% of the alendronate-treated group had one or more new vertebral fractures compared with 15.0% in the placebo-treated group. The risk of a new vertebral fracture was 47% lower in the alendronate-treated group compared with placebo. RR, relative risk. Data from Black DM, Cummings SR, Karpf DB et al. Randomized trial of effect of alendronate on risk of fracture in women with existing vertebral fractures. Lancet 1996; 348:1535–41.

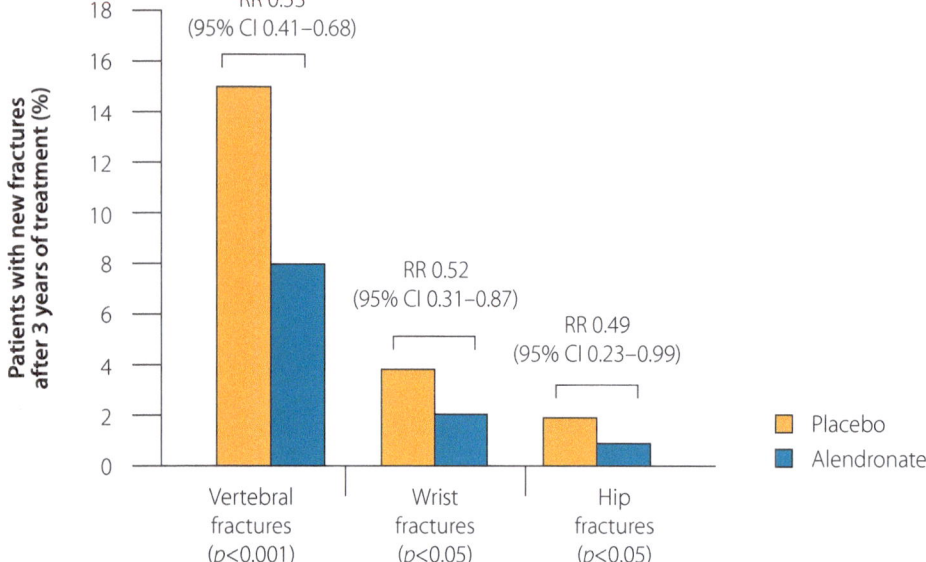

Effects of alendronate on bone mineral density

Figure 4.14. The effects of alendronate on bone mineral density (BMD) at the lumbar spine **(a)**, femoral neck **(b)**, and total hip **(c)** are shown. The Fracture Intervention Trial (FIT) included women aged 55–81 years with low femoral neck BMD with or without existing vertebral fractures. The women were randomly allocated to receive alendronate (5 mg/day increasing to 10 mg/day at 24 months), or placebo. There were significant increases in bone mass of 4.1% at femoral neck, 4.7% at total hip, and 6.2% at the lumbar spine with alendronate treatment as compared with placebo. There were also significant increases in BMD at other sites (trochanter, whole body, lateral spine, and proximal forearm). Reproduced with permission from Black DM, Cummings SR, Karpf DB et al. Randomized trial of effect of alendronate on risk of fracture in women with existing vertebral fractures. Lancet 1996; 348:1535–41.

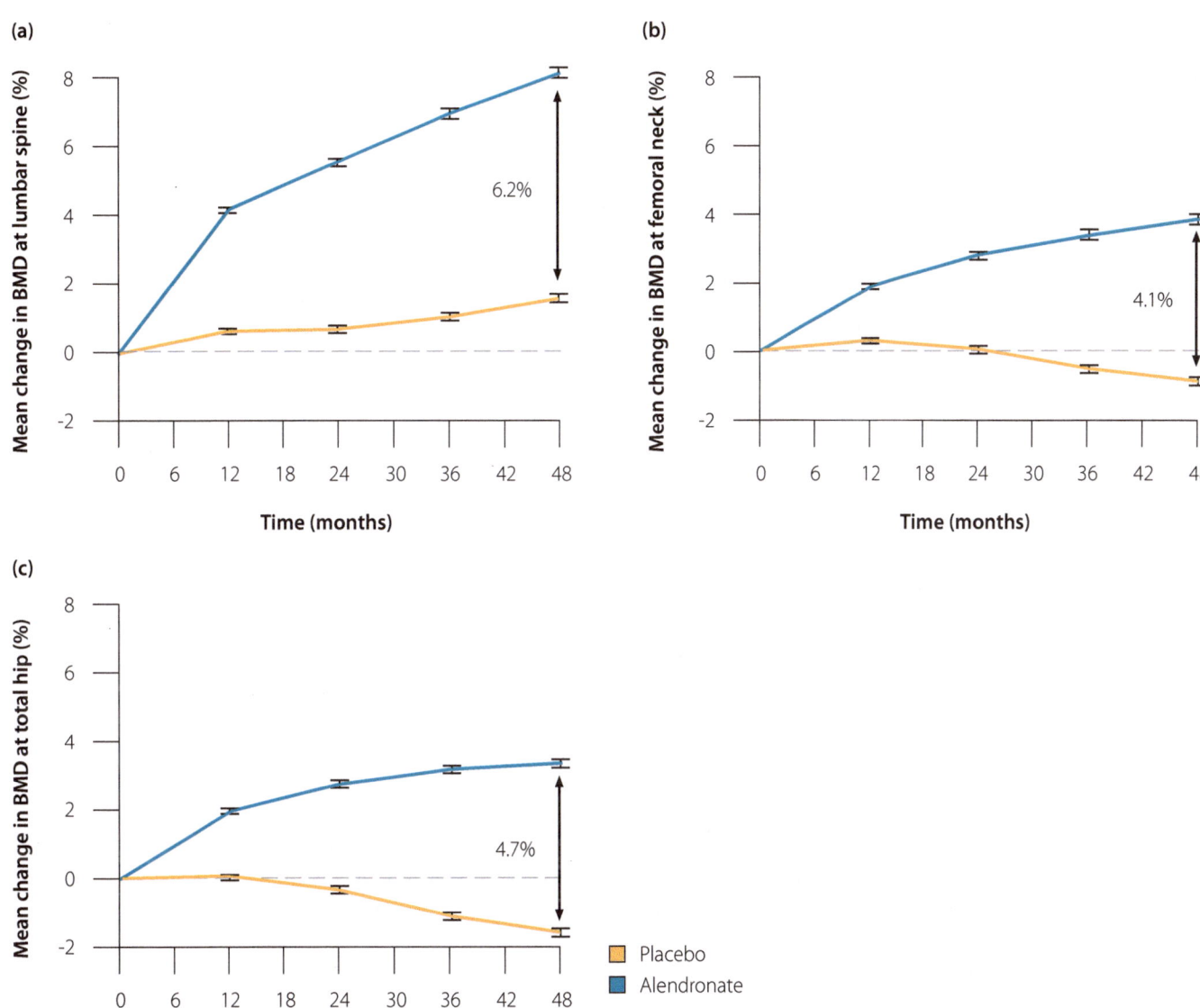

Effects of risedronate on incidence of new vertebral and nonvertebral fractures

Figure 4.15. The effects of risedronate on the incidence of new vertebral (**a**) and nonvertebral (**b**) fractures are shown. The study included 2458 postmenopausal women younger than 85 years of age who had at least one vertebral fracture at baseline. Over the study period, there was a significant reduction of 41% in the risk of new vertebral fractures in the risedronate group compared with the placebo group. For nonvertebral fractures the cumulative incidence over the study period was reduced by 39% in the risedronate group compared with placebo group. *$p<0.05$; †$p<0.01$; ‡$p<0.001$ versus placebo. RR, relative risk; CI, confidence interval. Adapted with permission from Harris ST, Watts NB, Genant HK et al. Effects of risedronate treatment on vertebral and nonvertebral fractures in women with postmenopausal osteoporosis. A randomized controlled trial. JAMA 1999; 282:1344–52.

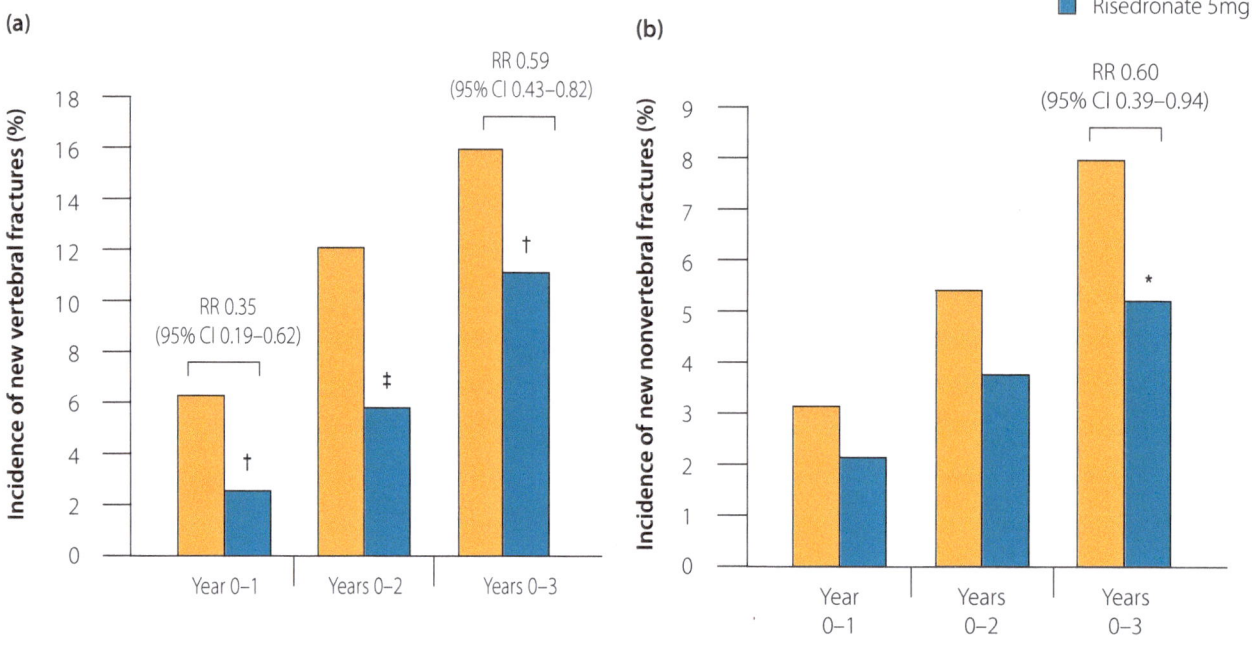

Effect of risedronate on incidence of hip fracture

Figure 4.16. The effect of risedronate on incidence of hip fracture is shown. The Hip Intervention Program (HIP) study included women 70–79 years of age who had low bone mineral density (BMD) at the femoral neck, and women 80 years or older who had at least one nonskeletal risk factor (eg, poor gait or a propensity to fall), or a low BMD at the femoral neck. The women were randomly allocated to receive risedronate (2.5 or 5 mg/day), or placebo. Overall, the incidence of hip fracture was 2.8% in the risedronate-treated group as compared with 3.9% in the placebo-treated group. For those aged 70–79 years the incidence of hip fracture was 1.9% in the risedronate-treated group compared with 3.2% in the placebo-treated group. Therefore, risedronate was shown to reduce the risk of hip fracture in women with confirmed osteoporosis, but not in those with risk factors other than low BMD. RR, relative risk; CI, confidence interval. Data from McClung MR, Geusens P, Miller PD et al. Effect of risedronate on the risk of hip fracture in elderly women. N Engl J Med 2001; 344:333–40.

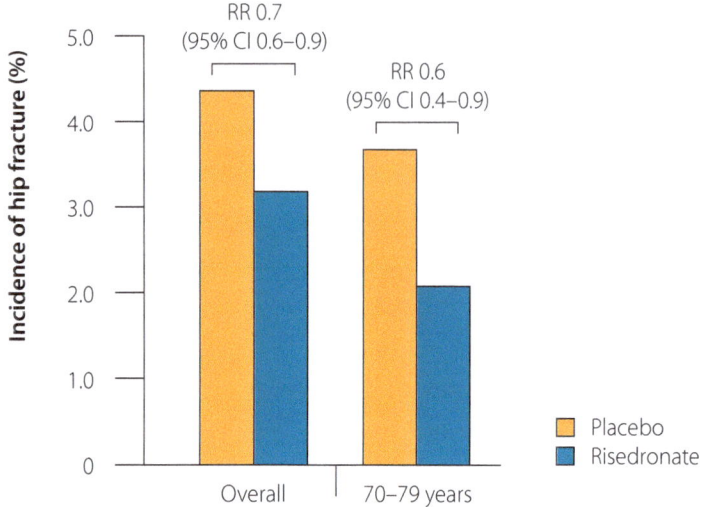

Effect of ibandronate on the incidence of vertebral fractures

Figure 4.17. The effect of ibandronate on the incidence of vertebral fractures is shown. The BONE study enrolled 2946 postmenopausal women with osteoporosis with a BMD T-score −2.0 at the lumbar spine in at least one vertebra and one to four prevalent vertebral fractures. Patients were randomized to receive placebo or oral ibandronate administered daily (2.5 mg/day) or intermittently (20 mg every other day for 12 doses every three months). The primary endpoint was the incidence of new vertebral fractures after three years. Overall the incidence of patients with new incident vertebral fractures at year 3 was estimated to be 9.6% (95% CI, 7.5–11.7) for the placebo group and 4.7% (95% CI, 3.2–6.2) and 4.9% (95% CI, 3.4–6.4) for the daily and intermittent ibandronate groups, respectively. Daily and intermittent oral ibandronate significantly reduced the risk of new vertebral fractures. No effect on nonvertebral fractures was demonstrated in the intention-to-treat (ITT) population. *$p<0.001$ versus placebo, †$p<0.0017$ versus placebo. RR, relative risk. Reproduced with permission from Chesnut CH 3rd, Skag A, Christiansen C; Oral Ibandronate Osteoporosis Vertebral Fracture Trial in North America and Europe (BONE). Effects of oral ibandronate administered daily or intermittently on fracture risk in postmenopausal osteoporosis. J Bone Miner Res 2004; 19:1241–9.

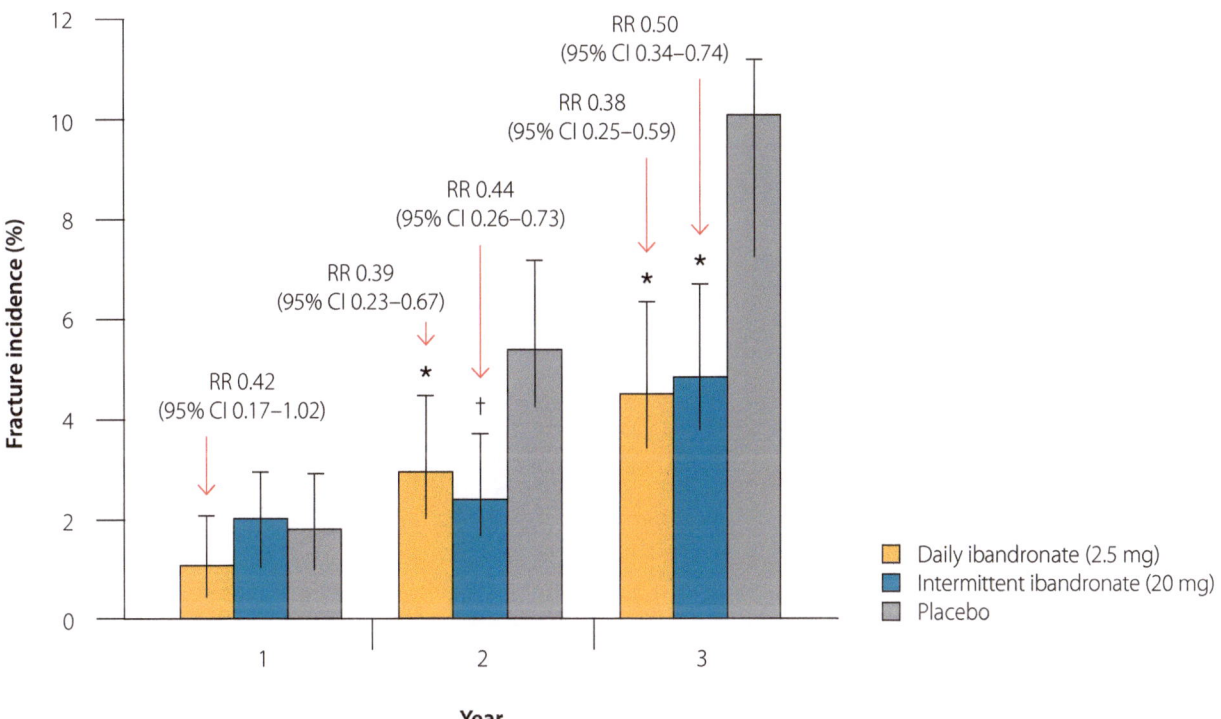

Calcitonin and vertebral fracture prevention

Figure 4.18. The effect of nasal calcitonin on the risk of vertebral fractures is shown. The Prevent Recurrence of Osteoporotic Fractures (PROOF) study included postmenopausal women with established osteoporosis who were randomly allocated to receive calcitonin (salmon calcitonin nasal spray 100, 200 or 400 IU/day), or placebo. The risk of new vertebral fractures was significantly decreased in the 200 IU calcitonin-treated group as compared with the placebo-treated group, but not with any of the other doses of calcitonin. Calcitonin had no effect on nonvertebral fractures. RR, relative risk; CI, confidence interval. Data from Chesnut CH 3rd, Silverman S, Andriano K et al. A randomized trial of nasal spray salmon calcitonin in postmenopausal women with established osteoporosis: the Prevent Recurrence of Osteoporotic Fractures Study. Am J Med 2000; 109:267–76.

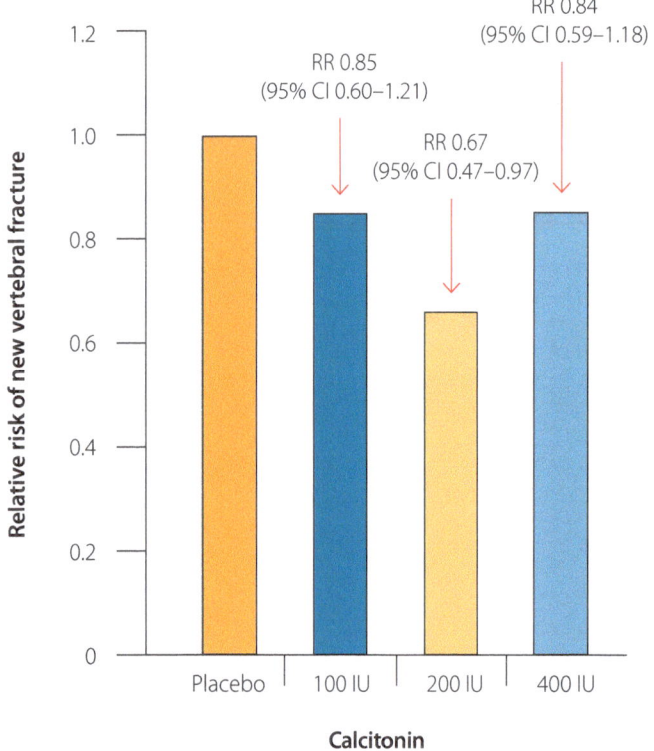

Structure of parathyroid hormone receptor

Figure 4.19. The parathyroid hormone receptor is a G-protein-coupled receptor that plays a major role in controlling the levels of calcium in the blood, and in bone formation. There are two stages of the interaction of parathyroid hormone (PTH) with its receptor: initially there is a docking interaction between the carboxy terminal portion of PTH 1–34 and the amino terminal extracellular domain of the receptor, and then the amino terminal portion of PTH can interact weakly with the juxtamembrane region of the receptor. Adapted with permission from Gardella TJ, Jüppner H. Molecular properties of the PTH/PTHrP receptor. Trends Endocrinol Metab 2001; 12:210–7.

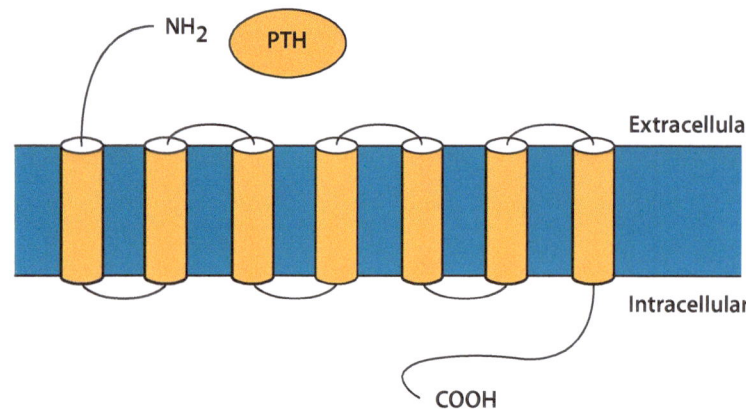

Effects of parathyroid hormone on bone mineral density

Figure 4.20. The effects of parathyroid hormone peptide 1–34 (PTH 1–34) on bone mineral density (BMD) at the lumbar spine, femoral neck, and total hip are shown. The study included postmenopausal women with prior vertebral fractures who were randomly allocated to receive PTH 1–34 (20 µg/day), or placebo. There was an increase in BMD at the lumbar spine of 9.7% in the PTH 1–34-treated group compared with 1.1% in the placebo-treated group, and an increase in BMD at the femoral neck of 2.8% in the PTH 1–34-treated group compared with a decrease of 0.7% in the placebo-treated group. The total hip BMD increased by 2.6% in the PTH 1–34-treated group and decreased by 1% in the placebo-treated group. Data from Neer RM, Arnaud CD, Zanchetta JR et al. Effect of parathyroid hormone (1–34) on fractures and bone mineral density in postmenopausal women with osteoporosis. N Engl J Med 2001; 344:1434–41.

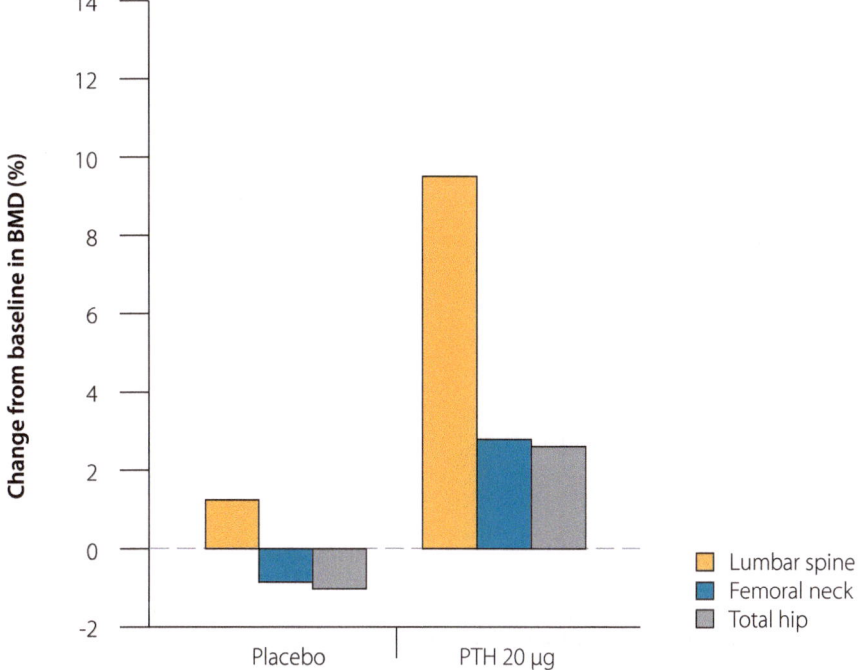

Effect of parathyroid hormone on incidence of new vertebral fractures

Figure 4.21. The effects of parathyroid hormone peptide 1–34 (PTH 1–34) on the risk of new vertebral fractures in women with postmenopausal osteoporosis and prior vertebral fracture. The women were randomly allocated to receive PTH 1–34, or placebo, administered subcutaneously once daily. The risk of one or more new vertebral fractures was reduced by 65% in the PTH 1–34-treated group as compared with placebo, the risk of two or more fractures by 77%, and the risk of at least one moderate or severe vertebral fracture by 90%. Treatment with PTH 1–34 also reduced the total number of vertebral fractures. *$p<0.001$ compared with placebo. RR, relative risk; CI, confidence interval. Data from Neer RM, Arnaud CD, Zanchetta JR et al. Effect of parathyroid hormone (1–34) on fractures and bone mineral density in postmenopausal women with osteoporosis. N Engl J Med 2001; 344:1434–41.

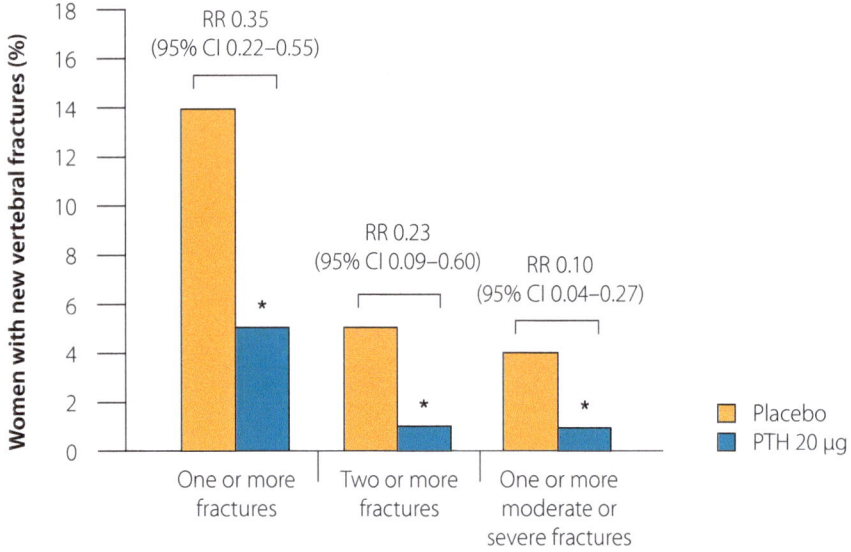

Effect of parathyroid hormone on incidence of new nonvertebral fractures and fragility fractures

Figure 4.22. The effects of parathyroid hormone peptide 1–34 (PTH 1–34) on new nonvertebral fractures and nonvertebral fragility fractures are shown. In the same patients as Figure 4.21, it was found that the incidence of one or more new nonvertebral fractures was 10% in the placebo-treated group and 6% in the PTH 1–34-treated group and the incidence of fragility fractures 6% and 3%, respectively. Some of the women had a new fracture at more than one skeletal site or had more than one new fracture at the same site (eg, in both extremities). *$p=0.04$; †$p=0.02$ compared with placebo. RR, relative risk; CI, confidence interval. Adapted from Neer RM, Arnaud CD, Zanchetta JR, et al. Effect of parathyroid hormone (1–34) on fractures and bone mineral density in postmenopausal women with osteoporosis. N Engl J Med 2001; 344:1434–41.

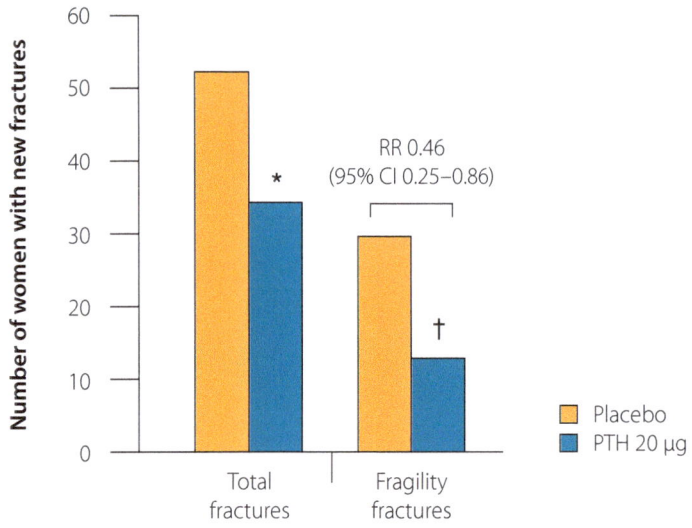

Effect of strontium ranelate on bone mineral density

Figure 4.23. The effects of strontium ranelate on bone mineral density (BMD) at the lumbar spine **(a)**, femoral neck **(b)**, and total hip **(c)** over a 3-year period versus placebo are shown. BMD increased continuously in the strontium ranelate-treated group over the 3-year period, with no trend toward a plateau. At 3 years, the BMD in the strontium ranelate-treated group had increased by 14.4% at the lumbar spine, 8.3% at the femoral neck, and 9.8% at the total hip, compared with placebo. Reproduced with permission from Meunier PJ, Roux C, Seeman E et al. The effects of strontium ranelate on the risk of vertebral fracture in women with postmenopausal osteoporosis. N Engl J Med 2004; 350:459–68.

(a) Lumbar spine

(b) Femoral neck

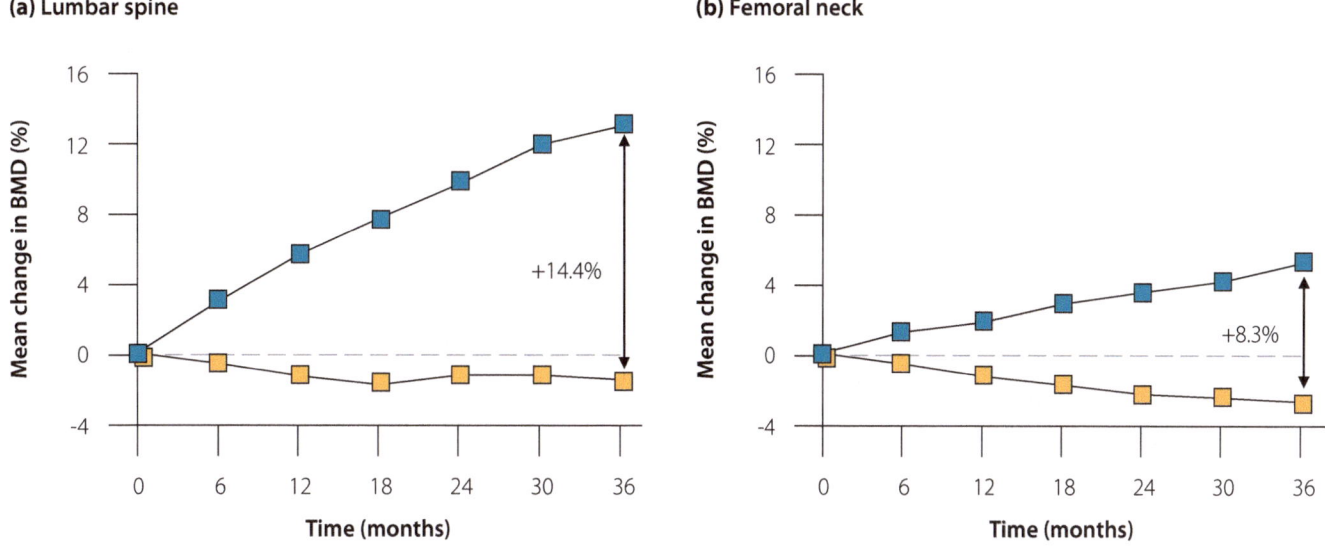

(c) Total hip

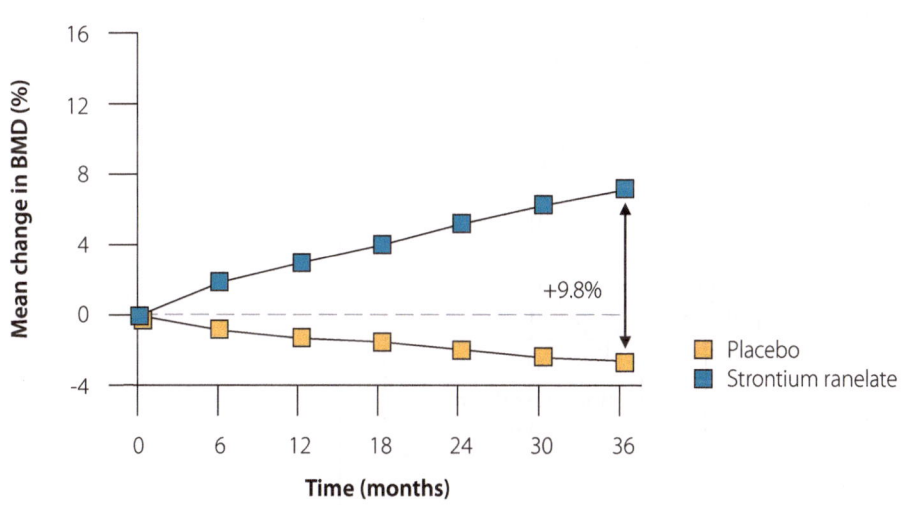

Mode of action of strontium ranelate

Figure 4.24. Strontium ranelate has a unique dual action on bone metabolism as it appears to simultaneously increase bone formation and decrease bone resorption. Strontium ranelate has been shown *in vitro* to increase bone formation by increasing the replication of preosteoblasts (Pre-OBs) into osteoblasts (OBs), leading to an increase in bone matrix synthesis. It has also been shown to decrease bone resorption by reducing the differentiation of pre-osteoclasts (Pre-OCs) into osteoclasts (OCs), and the bone resorbing activity of osteoclasts. The bone created with the use of strontium ranelate is lamellar (ie, normal) and well mineralized. Bone strength is also increased as a result of improvements in the bone biomechanical properties. From Marie PJ, Ammann P, Boivin G et al. Mechanisms of action and therapeutic potential of strontium in bone. Calcif Tissue Int 2001; 69:121–9.

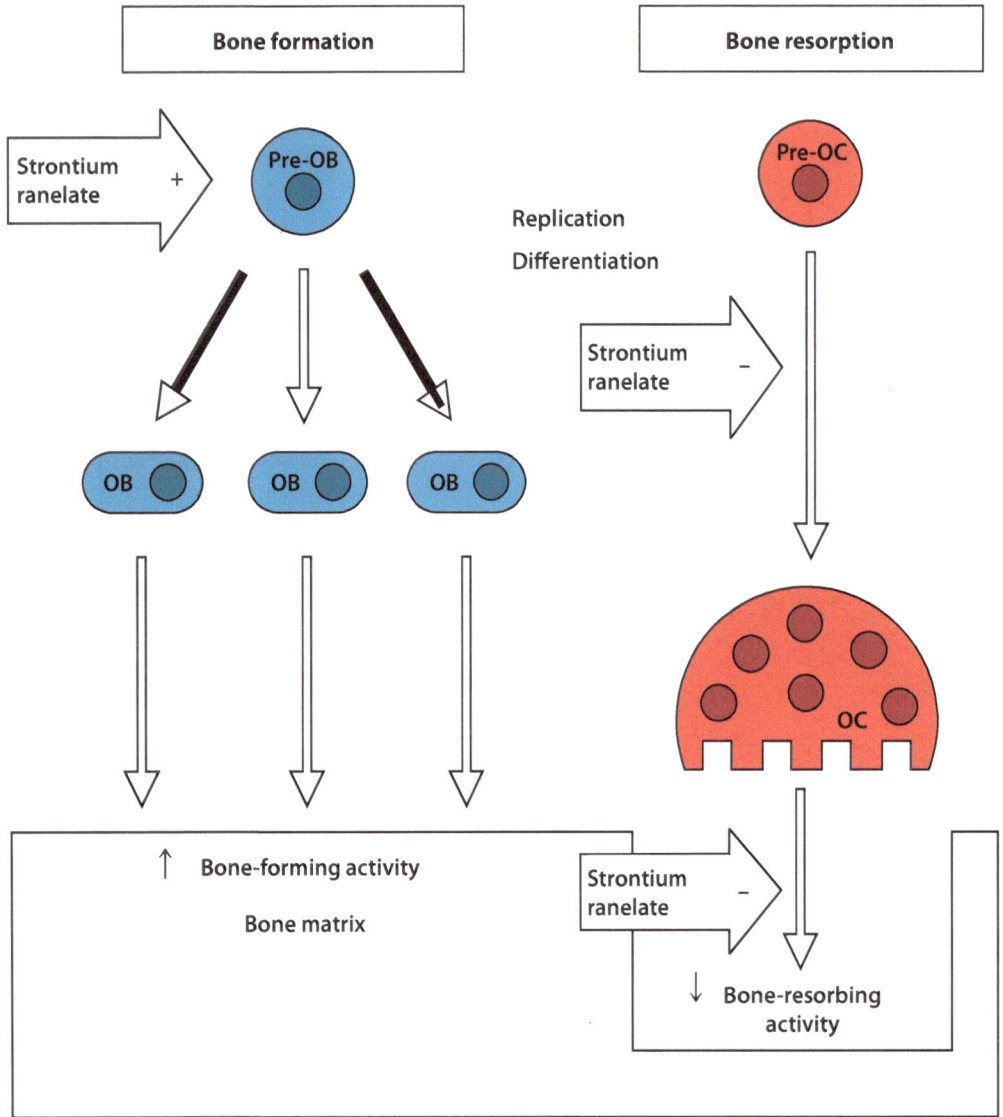

Effect of strontium ranelate on vertebral fracture risk

Figure 4.25. The Spinal Osteoporosis Therapeutic Intervention (SOTI) trial was a randomized, double-blind, placebo-controlled trial, evaluating the efficacy of strontium ranelate 2 g/day orally, to reduce the incidence of patients experiencing a new vertebral fracture(s) during a 3-year treatment period, each group receiving in addition calcium and vitamin D. Postmenopausal women (mean age ± SD 69.7 ± 7.3 years) were included in two parallel groups. Lumbar bone mineral density was significantly increased by 14.4% compared with placebo ($p<0.001$) at 3 years. The vertebral antifracture efficacy of strontium ranelate was demonstrated with reductions in the relative risk (RR) of 49% after 1 year of treatment ($p<0.001$), and 41% ($p<0.001$) after 3 years in the strontium ranelate-treated group compared with the placebo-treated group. CI, confidence interval. Adapted with permission from Meunier PJ, Roux C, Seeman E et al. The effects of strontium ranelate on the risk of vertebral fracture in women with postmenopausal osteoporosis. N Engl J Med 2004; 350:459–68.

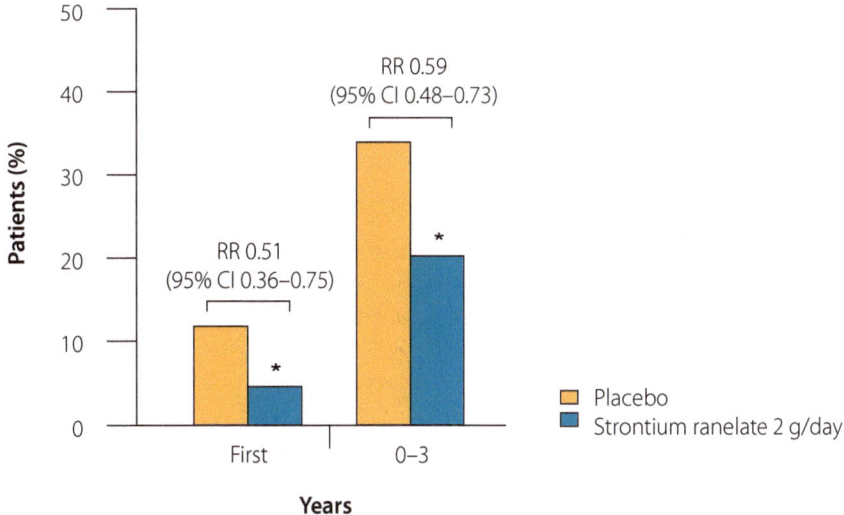

Effect of strontium ranelate on hip fractures

Figure 4.26. The TReatment Of Peripheral OSteoporosis (TROPOS) trial was a randomized, double-blind, placebo-controlled trial, evaluating the efficacy of strontium ranelate 2 g/day orally, to reduce the number of patients experiencing nonvertebral fracture(s) during a 3-year treatment period. Each group received additional calcium and vitamin D. Postmenopausal women were included in two parallel groups. Femoral neck and total hip bone mineral density increased by 8.2% and 9.8% respectively compared with placebo ($p<0.001$) at 3 years. The nonvertebral antifracture efficacy of strontium ranelate was demonstrated with a significant reduction in the relative risk (RR) over 3 years in the strontium ranelate-treated group compared with the placebo-treated group ($p<0.05$). In patients aged 74 years and over with a T-score of −2.5, the RR of hip fracture was significantly reduced by 36% over 3 years in the strontium ranelate-treated group compared with the placebo-treated group ($p<0.05$). Data from Reginster JY, Seeman E, De Vernejoul MC et al. Strontium ranelate reduces the risk of nonvertebral fractures in postmenopausal women with osteoporosis: treatment of peripheral osteoporosis (TROPOS) study. J Clin Endocrinol Metab 2005; 90:2816–22.

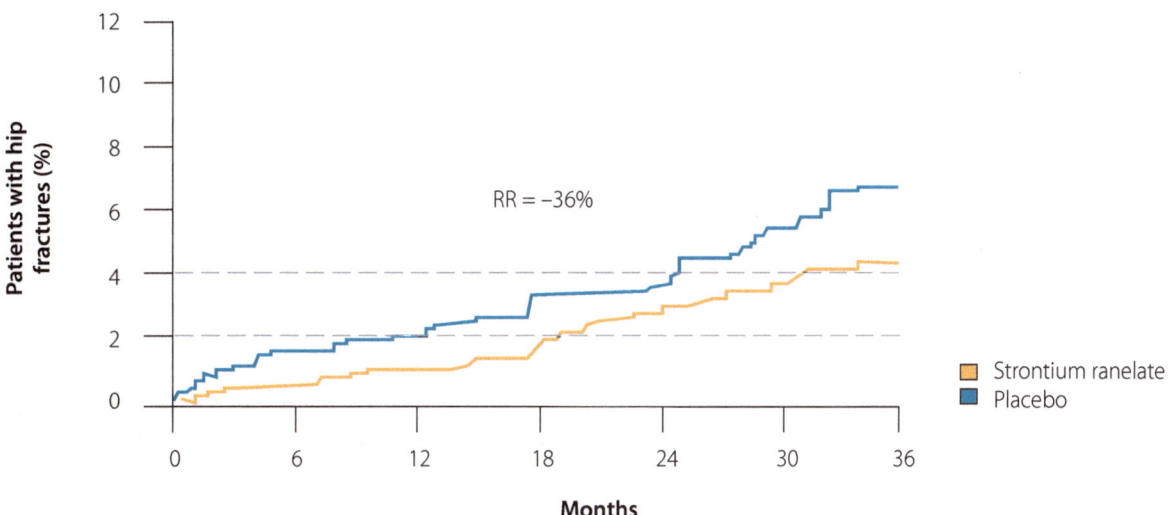

References

Adami S, Giannini S, Bianchi G et al. Vitamin D status and response to treatment in post-menopausal osteoporosis. Osteoporos Int 2009; 20:239–44.

American Association of Clinical Endocrinologists. Medical guidelines for clinical practice for the prevention and treatment of postmenopausal osteoporosis: 2001 edition, with selected updates for 2003. Endocr Pract 2003; 9:544–64.

Avenell A, Gillespie WJ, Gillespie LD et al. Vitamin D and vitamin D analogues for preventing fractures associated with involutional and post-menopausal osteoporosis. Cochrane Database Syst Rev 2005; 18:CD001880.

Banciu M, Marza F, Ben Hadid R et al. Recent findings on the role of physical exercise in osteoporosis. Osteoporos Int 2005; 16:187.

Baron R, Tsouderos Y. In vitro effects of S12911-2 on osteoclast function and bone marrow macrophage differentiation. Eur J Pharmacol 2002; 450:11–7.

Barrett-Connor E, Grady D, Sashegyi A et al. Raloxifene and cardiovascular events in osteoporotic women: four-year results from the MORE (Multiple Outcomes of Raloxifene Evaluation) randomized trial. JAMA 2002; 287:847–57.

Beral V, Million Women Study Collaborators. Breast cancer and hormone-replacement therapy in the Million Women Study. Lancet 2003; 362:419–27.

Bischoff-Ferrari HA. How to select the doses of vitamin D in the management of osteoporosis. Osteoporos Int 2007; 18:401–7.

Bischoff-Ferrari HA, Willett WC, Wong JB et al. Fracture prevention with vitamin D supplementation. JAMA 2005; 293:2257–64.

Black DM, Cummings SR, Karpf DB et al. Randomised trial of effect of alendronate on risk of fracture in women with existing vertebral fractures. Lancet 1996; 348:1535–41.

Black DM, Delmas PD, Eastell R et al. Once-yearly zoledronic acid for treatment of postmenopausal osteoporosis. N Engl J Med 2007; 356:1809–22.

Black DM, Schwartz AV, Ensrud KE et al. Effects of continuing or stopping alendronate after 5 years of treatment: the Fracture Intervention Trial Long-term Extension (FLEX): a randomized trial. JAMA 2006; 296:2927–38.

Bone HG, Bolognese MA, Yuen CK et al. Effects of denosumab on bone mineral density and bone turnover in postmenopausal women. J Clin Endocrinol Metab 2008; 93:2149–57.

Bone HG, Hosking D, Devogelaer JP et al. Ten years experience with alendronate for osteoporosis in postmenopausal women. N Engl J Med 2004; 350:1189–99.

Bonnelye E, Chabadel A, Saltel F et al. Dual effect of strontium ranelate: stimulation of osteoblast differentiation and inhibition of osteoclast formation and resorption in vitro. Bone 2008; 42:129–38.

Boonen S, McClung M, Eastell R et al. Safety and efficacy of risedronate in reducing fracture risk in osteoporotic women aged 80 and older: implications for the use of antiresorptive agents in the old and oldest old. J Am Geriatr Soc 2004; 52:1832–9.

Boonen S, Lips P, Bouillon R et al. Need for additional calcium to reduce the risk of hip fracture with vitamin D supplementation: evidence from a comparative meta-analysis of randomized controlled trials. J Clin Endocrinol Metab. 2007; 92:1415–23.

Brown JP, Josse RG. 2002 clinical practice guidelines for the diagnosis and management of osteoporosis in Canada. CMAJ 2002; 167(Suppl 10):S1–S34.

Bruyère O, Malaise, Neuprez A et al. European postmenopausal women have high prevalence of vitamin D inadequacy. Arthritis Rheum 2006; 54:S585.

Bruyere O, Roux C, Detilleux J et al. Relationship between bone mineral density changes and fracture risk reduction in patients treated with strontium ranelate. J Clin Endocrinol Metab. 2007; 92:3076–81.

Canalis E, Hott M, Deloffre P et al. The divalent strontium salt S12911 enhances bone cell replication and bone formation in vitro. Bone 1996; 18:517–23.

Cauley JA, Robbins J, Chen Z et al. Effects of estrogen plus progestin on risk of fracture and bone mineral density. The Women's Health Initiative Randomized Trial. JAMA 2003; 290:1729–38.

Chapuy MC, Arlot ME, Duboeuf F et al. Vitamin D3 and calcium to prevent hip fractures in the elderly women. N Engl J Med 1992; 327:1637–42.

Chapuy MC, Pamphile R, Paris E et al. Combined calcium and vitamin D3 supplementation in elderly women: confirmation of reversal of secondary hyperparathyroidism and hip fracture risk: the Decalyos II study. Osteoporos Int 2002; 13:257–64.

Chesnut CH 3rd, Silverman S, Andriano K et al. A randomised trial of nasal spray salmon calcitonin in postmenopausal women with established osteoporosis: the Prevent Recurrence of Osteoporotic Fractures Study. Am J Med 2000; 109:267–76.

Chesnut III CH, Skag A, Christiansen C. Oral Ibandronate Osteoporosis Vertebral Fracture Trial in North America and Europe (BONE). Effects of oral ibandronate administered daily or intermittently on fracture risk in postmenopausal osteoporosis. J Bone Miner Res 2004; 19:1241–9.

Choi HJ, Im JA, Kim SH. Changes in bone markers after once-weekly low-dose alendronate in postmenopausal women with moderate bone loss. Maturitas 2008; 60:170–6.

Cranney A, Tugwell P, Adachi J et al. Meta-analyses of therapies for postmenopausal osteoporosis. III. Meta-analysis of risedronate for the treatment of postmenopausal women. Endocr Rev 2002a; 23:517–23.

Cranney A, Wells G, Willan A et al. Meta-analyses of therapies for postmenopausal osteoporosis. II. Meta-analysis of alendronate for the treatment of postmenopausal women. Endocr Rev 2002b; 23:508–16.

Cranney A, Wells GA, Yetisir E et al. Ibandronate for the prevention of nonvertebral fractures: a pooled analysis of individual patient data. Osteoporos Int 2009; 20:291–7.

Cummings SR, Black DM, Thompson DE et al. Effect of alendronate on risk of fracture in women with low bone density but without vertebral fractures. JAMA 1998; 280:2077–82.

Cummings SR, Ettinger B, Delmas PD et al. The effects of tibolone in older postmenopausal women. N Engl J Med 2008; 359:697–708.

Cummings SR, San Martin J, McClung MR et al. FREEDOM Trial. Denosumab for prevention of fractures in postmenopausal women with osteoporosis. N Engl J Med 2009; 361:756–65.

Dawson-Hughes B, Heaney RP, Holick MF et al. Estimates of optimal vitamin D status. Osteoporos Int 2005; 16:713–6.

Delmas PD. Treatment of postmenopausal osteoporosis. Lancet 2002; 359:2018–26.

Delmas PD, Adami S, Strugala C et al. Intravenous ibandronate injections in postmenopausal women with osteoporosis: one-year results from the Dosing Intravenous Administration Study. Arthritis Rheum 2006a; 54:1838–46.

Delmas PD, Bjarnason NH, Mitlak BH et al. Effects of raloxifene on bone mineral density, serum cholesterol concentrations, and uterine endometrium in postmenopausal women. N Engl J Med 1997; 337:1641–7.

Delmas PD, Ensrud KE, Adachi JD et al. Efficacy of raloxifene on vertebral fracture risk reduction in postmenopausal women with osteoporosis: four-year results from a randomized clinical trial. J Clin Endocrinol Metab 2002; 87:3609–17.

Delmas PD, Genant HK, Crans GG et al. Severity of prevalent vertebral fractures and the risk of subsequent vertebral and nonvertebral fractures: results from the MORE trial. Bone 2003; 33:522–32.

Delmas PD, Licata AA, Reginster JY et al. Fracture Risk reduction during treatment with teriparatide is independent of pre-treatment bone turnover. Bone 2006b; 39:237–43.

Delmas PD, Recker RR, Chesnut CH 3rd et al. Daily and intermittent oral ibandronate normalize bone turnover and provide significant reduction in vertebral fracture risk: results from the BONE study. Osteoporos Int 2004; 15:792–8.

Eastell R. Treatment of postmenopausal osteoporosis. N Engl J Med 1998; 338:736–46.

Egger P, Duggleby S, Hobbs R et al. Cigarette smoking and bone mineral density in the elderly. J Epidemiol Community Health 1996; 50:47–50.

Ernst E. Exercise for female osteoporosis. A systematic review of randomised clinical trials. Sports Med 1998; 25:359–68.

European Medicines Agency (EMEA): London. Question and answers on the safety of Protelos/Osseor (strontium ranelate). 2007. Ref. EMEA/534613/2007. Available at: www.emea.europa.eu/humandocs/PDFs/ EPAR/protelos/Protelos_Q&A_53461307en.pdf. Accessed October 1, 2008.

Ettinger B, Black DM, Mitlak BH et al. Reduction of vertebral fracture risk in postmenopausal women with osteoporosis treated with raloxifene: results from a 3-year randomized clinical trial. JAMA 1999; 282:637–45.

Gardella TJ, Jüppner H. Molecular properties of the PTH/PTHrP receptor. Trends Endocrinol Metab 2001; 12:210–7.

Going S, Lohman T, Houtkooper L et al. Effects of exercise on bone mineral density in calcium-replete postmenopausal women with and without hormone replacement therapy. Osteoporos Int 2003; 14:637–643.

Greenspan SL, Bone HG, Ettinger MP et al. Effect of recombinant human parathyroid hormone (1-84) on vertebral fracture and bone mineral density in postmenopausal women with osteoporosis: a randomized trial. Annals Int Med 2007; 146:326–39.

Grosso A, Douglas I, Hingorani A et al. Post-marketing assessment of the safety of strontium ranelate; a novel case-only approach to the early detection of adverse drug reactions. Br J Clin Pharmacol 2008; 66:689–94.

Hansen MA, Overgaard K, Riis BJ et al. Potential risk factors for development of postmenopausal osteoporosis—examined over a 12-year period. Osteoporos Int 1991; 1:95–102.

Harris ST, Blumentals WA, Miller PD. Ibandronate and the risk of non-vertebral and clinical fractures in women with postmenopausal osteoporosis: results of a meta-analysis of phase III studies. Curr Med Res Opin 2008; 24:237–45.

Harris ST, Watts NB, Genant HK et al. Effects of risedronate treatment on vertebral and nonvertebral fractures in women with postmenopausal osteoporosis. A randomised controlled trial. JAMA 1999; 282:1344–52.

Heikinheimo RJ, Inkovaara JA, Harju EJ et al. Annual injection of vitamin D and fractures of aged bones. Calcif Tissue Int 1992; 51:105–10.

Hodsman AB, Bauer DC, Dempster DW et al. Parathyroid hormone and teriparatide for the treatment of osteoporosis: a review of the evidence and suggested guidelines for its use. Endo Rev 2005; 26:688–703.

Hodsman AB, Hanley, Ettinger MP et al. Efficacy and safety of human parathyroid hormone (1-84) in increasing bone mineral density in postmenopausal osteoporosis. J Clin End Metab 2003; 88:5212–20.

Hotta M, Shibasaki T, Sato K et al. The importance of body weight history in the occurrence and recovery of osteoporosis in patients with anorexia nervosa: evaluation by dual X-ray absorptiometry and bone metabolic markers. Eur J Endocrinol 1998; 139:276–83.

Hurtel Lemaire AS, Mentaverri R, Caudrillier A et al. The calcium-sensing receptor is involved in strontium ranelate-induced osteoclast apoptosis. New insights into the associated signaling pathways. J Biol Chem 2009; 284:575–84.

Jilka RL, Weinstein RS, Bellido T et al. Increased bone formation by prevention of osteoblast apoptosis with parathyroid hormone. J Clin Invest 1999; 104:371–373.

Kanis JA, Burlet N, Cooper C et al. European guidance for the diagnosis and management of osteoporosis in postmenopausal women. Osteoporos Int 2008; 19:399–428.

Kiel DP, Baron JA, Anderson JJ et al. Smoking eliminates the protective effect of oral estrogens on the risk for hip fracture among women. Ann Intern Med 1992; 116:716–21.

Lau E, Papaioannou A, Dolovich L et al. Patients' adherence to osteoporosis therapy: exploring the perceptions of postmenopausal women. Can Fam Physician 2008; 54:394–402.

Lewiecki EM, Keaveny TM, Kopperdahl D et al. Once-monthly oral Ibandronate improves biomechanical determinants of bone strength in women with postmenopausal osteoporosis. J Clin Endocrinol Metab 2009; 94:171–80.

Lindsay R, Scheels WH, Neer R et al. Sustained vertebral fracture risk reduction after withdrawal of teriparatide (recombinant human parathyroid hormone (1–34)) in postmenopausal women with osteoporosis. Arch Intern Med 2004; 164:2024–30.

Lyles KW, Colon-Emeric CS, Magaziner JS et al. Zoledronic acid and clinical fractures and mortality after hip fracture. N Engl J Med 2007; 357:1799–1809.

Malabanan A, Veronikis IE, Holick MF. Redefining vitamin D insufficiency. Lancet 1998; 351:805–6.

Marcus R, Wang O, Satterwhite J et al. The skeletal response to teriparatide is largely independent of age, initial bone mineral density, and prevalent vertebral fractures in postmenopausal women with osteoporosis. J Bone Miner Res 2003; 18:18–23.

Marie PJ, Ammann P, Boivin G et al. Mechanisms of action and therapeutical potential of strontium in bone. Calcif Tissue Int 2001; 69:121–129.

Martino S, Cauley JA, Barrett-Connor E et al; CORE Investigators. Continuing outcomes relevant to Evista: breast cancer incidence in postmenopausal osteoporotic women in a randomized trial of raloxifene. J Natl Cancer Inst 2004; 96:1751–61.

Mashiba T, Hirano T, Turner CH et al. Suppressed bone turnover by bisphosphonates increases microdamage accumulation and reduces some biomechanical properties in dog rib. J Bone Miner Res 2000; 15:613–20.

Mastaglia SR, Pellegrini GG, Mandalunis PM et al. Vitamin D insufficiency reduces the protective effect of bisphosphonate on ovariectomy-induced bone loss in rats. Bone 2006; 39:837–44.

McClung MR. Bisphosphonates. Endcrinol Metab Clin North Am 2003; 32:253–71.

McClung MR, Geusens P, Miller PD et al. Effect of risedronate on the risk of hip fracture in elderly women. N Engl J Med 2001; 344:333–40.

McClung MR, Lewiecki EM, Cohen SB et al. Denosumab in postmenopausal women with low bone mineral density. N Engl J Med 2006; 354:821–31.

Meunier PJ, Roux C, Seeman E et al. The effects of strontium ranelate on the risk of vertebral fracture in women with postmenopausal osteoporosis. N Engl J Med 2004; 350:459–68.

Miller PD, Bolognese MA, Lewiecki EM et al. Effect of denosumab on bone density and turnover in postmenopausal women with low bone mass after long-term continued, discontinued, and restarting of therapy: a randomized blinded phase 2 clinical trial. Bone 2008; 43:222–9.

Mundy GR. Osteoporosis: pathophysiology and nonpharmacological management. Best Pract Res Clin Rheumatol 2001; 15:727–45.

Neer RM, Arnaud CD, Zanchetta JR et al. Effect of parathyroid hormone (I-34) on fractures and bone mineral density in postmenopausal women with osteoporosis. N Engl J Med 2001; 344:1434–41.

Neuprez A, Reginster JY. Bone-forming agents in the management of osteoporosis. Best Practice & Research Clinical Endocrinology & Metabolism 2008; 22:869–83.

Prince RL, Devine A, Dhaliwal SS et al. Effects of calcium supplementation on clinical fracture and bone structure. Arch Intern Med 2006; 166:869–75.

Prince R, Sipos A, Hossain A et al. Sustained nonvertebral fragility fracture risk reduction after discontinuation of teriparatide treatment. J Bone Miner Res 2005; 20:1507–13.

Rabenda V, Vanoverloop J, Fabri V et al. Low incidence of anti-osteoporosis treatment after hip fracture. J Bone Joint Surg Am 2008; 90:2142–8.

Reginster JY, Adami S, Lakatos P et al. Efficacy and tolerability of once-monthly oral ibandronate in postmenopausal osteoprosis: 2-year results from the MOBILE study. Ann Rheum Dis 2006; 65:654–61.

Reginster JY, Deroisy R, Lecart MP et al. A double-blind, placebo-controlled, dose-finding trial of intermittent nasal salmon calcitonin for prevention of postmenopausal lumbar spine bone loss. Am J Med 1995; 98:452–8.

Reginster JY, Felsenberg D, Boonen S et al. Effects of long-term strontium ranelate treatment on the risk of nonvertebral and vertebral fractures in postmenopausal osteoporosis: Results of a five-year, randomized, placebo-controlled trial. Arthritis Rheum 2008a; 58:1687–95.

Reginster JY, Franchimont P. Side effect of SSCT given by intranasal spray compared with intra-muscular injection. Clin Exp Rheumatol 1985; 3:155–7.

Reginster JY, Malaise O, Neuprez A et al. Strontium ranelate in the prevention of osteoporotic fractures. Int J Clin Pract 2007; 61:324–8.

Reginster JY, Minne HW, Sorensen OH et al. Randomized trial of the effects of risedronate on vertebral fractures in women with established postmenopausal osteoporosis. Osteoporos Int 2000; 11:83–91.

Reginster JY, Sawicki A, Roces-Varela et al. Long-term treatment of postmenopausal osteoporosis with strontium ranelate: results at 8 years. Bone 2009; in press.

Reginster JY, Seeman E, De Vernejoul MC et al. Strontium ranelate reduces the risk of nonvertebral fractures in postmenopausal women with osteoporosis: treatment of peripheral osteoporosis (TROPOS) study. J Clin Endocrinol Metab 2005; 90:2816–22.

Reginster JY, Spector T, Badurski J et al. A short-term run-in study can significantly contribute to increasing the quality of long-term osteoporosis trials. The strontium ranelate phase III program. Osteoporos Int 2002; 13(S1):S30.

Reginster JY, Taquet AN, Fraikin G et al. Parathyroid hormone in the treatment of involutional osteoporosis: back to the future. Osteoporos Int 1997; 7:S163–7.

Reid DM, Hosking D, Kendler D et al. A comparison of the effect of alendronate and risedronate on bone mineral density in postmenopausal women with osteoporosis: 24-month results from FACTS-International. Int J Clin Pract 2008; 62:575–84.

Riggs BL, Hartmann LC. Selective estrogen-receptor modulators — mechanisms of action and application to clinical practice. N Engl J Med 2003; 348:618–29.

Rizzoli R, Boonen S, Brandi ML et al. The role of calcium and vitamin D in the management of osteoporosis. Bone 2008a; 42:246–9.

Rizzoli R, Burlet N, Cahall D et al. Osteonecrosis of the jaw and bisphosphonates treatment for osteoporosis. Bone 2008b; 42:841–7.

Rossouw JE, Anderson GL, Prentice RL et al. Risks and benefits of estrogen plus progestin in healthy postmenopausal women: principal results from the Women's Health Initiative randomized controlled trial. JAMA 2002; 288:321–33.

Roux C, Reginster JY, Fechtenbaum J et al. Vertebral fracture risk reduction with strontium ranelate in women with postmenopausal osteoporosis is independent of baseline risk factors. J Bone Miner Res 2006; 21:536–42.

Rubin MR, Bilezikian JP. New anabolic therapies in osteoporosis. Endocrinol Metab Clin North Am 2003; 32:285–307.

Sahota O, Mundey MK, San P et al. The relationship between vitamin D and parathyroid hormone: calcium homeostasis, bone turnover, and bone mineral density in postmenopausal women with established osteoporosis. Bone 2004; 35:312–9.

Seeman E, Devogelaer J, Lorenc R et al. Strontium ranelate reduces the risk of vertebral fractures in patients with osteopenia. J Bone Miner Res 2008; 23:433–8.

Seeman E, Vellas B, Benhamou C et al. Strontium ranelate reduces the risk of vertebral and nonvertebral fractures in women eighty years of age and older. J Bone Miner Res 2006; 21:1113–20.

Shea B, Wells G, Cranney A et al. Osteoporosis Methodology Group; Osteoporosis Research Advisory Group. Calcium supplementation on bone loss in postmenopausal women. Cochrane Database Syst Rev 2004;(1):CD004526.

Shea B, Wells G, Cranney A et al. Meta-analysis of calcium supplementation for the prevention of postmenopausal osteoporosis. Endocrine Reviews 2002; 23:552–9.

Shrader SP, Ragucci KR. Parathyroid hormone (1-84) and treatment of osteoporosis. Annals Pharmacotherapy 2005; 39:1511–6.

Silverman SL, Watts NB, Delmas PD et al. Effectiveness of bisphosphonates on nonvertebral and hip fractures in the first year of therapy: the risedronate and alendronate (REAL) cohort Study. Osteoporos Int 2007; 18:25–34.

Suzuki A, Sekiguchi S, Asano S et al. Pharmacological topics of bone metabolism: recent advances in pharmacological management of osteoporosis. J Pharmacol Sci 2008; 106:530–5.

Takahashi N, Sasaki T, Tsouderos Y et al. S 12911-2 inhibits osteoclastic bone resorption in vitro. J Bone Miner Res 2003; 18:1082–7.

Tilyard MW, Spears GF, Thomson J et al. Treatment of postmenopausal osteoporosis with calcitriol or calcium. N Engl J Med 1992; 326:357–62.

Torgerson DJ, Bell-Syer SE. Hormone replacement therapy and prevention of nonvertebral fractures. A meta-analysis of randomised trials. JAMA 2001a; 285:2891–7.

Torgerson DJ, Bell-Syer SE. Hormone replacement therapy and prevention of vertebral fractures: a meta-analysis of randomised trials. BMC Musculoskelet Disord 2001b; 2:7.

Tosteson AN, Burge RT, Marshall DA et al. Therapies for treatment of osteoporosis in US women: cost-effectiveness and budget impact considerations. Am J Manag Care 2008; 14:605–15.

Ward KD, Klesges RC. A meta-analysis of the effects of cigarette smoking on bone mineral density. Calcif Tissue Int 2001; 68:259–70.

Watts NB. Bisphosphonate treatment of osteoporosis. Clin Geriatr Med 2003; 19:395–414.

Watts NB. Bisphosphonate treatment for osteoporosis. In: The Osteoporotic Syndrome. Edited by LV Avioli. San Diego: Academic Press, 2000;121–32.

Wehren LE. The epidemiology of osteoporosis and fractures in geriatric medicine. Clin Geriatr Med 2003; 19:245–58.

Winner SJ, Morgan CA, Evans JG. Perimenopausal risk of falling and incidence of distal forearm fracture. BMJ 1989; 298:1486–8.

Woodis CB. Once-yearly administered intravenous zoledronic acid for postmenopausal osteoporosis. Ann Pharmacother 2008; 42:1085–9.

Chapter 5
Conclusion

René Rizzoli

With the trend towards increased life expectancy, a women is likely to live more than one-third of her life in the state of sex hormone deficiency which characterizes menopause. At the age of 50, one out of two women is at risk of experiencing a fracture during the rest of her life, with the consequences of pain, long-term incapacity and increased mortality. Over the last few years it has become clear that despite a positive effect on the prevention of postmenopausal osteoporosis and on the associated risk of fracture, hormone replacement therapy can not be considered for the long-term prevention of postmenopausal osteoporosis, because the higher risk of side effects makes the risk/benefit ratio rather unfavorable.

Under these conditions, one could ask the question whether osteoporotic fractures would not be the price to pay as a consequence of increased life expectancy. After going through the information presented in this book, and looking at the pathophysiology, epidemiology, prevention and treatment of osteoporosis, I very much hope that you will join me in answering 'no' to this question. This message may seem rather optimistic. However, we are now beginning to understand the pathophysiology of the disease and identify risk factors for osteoporosis. We have reliable and performant tools capable of diagnosing the disease before the occurrence of its complication that represents a fracture. The major role of bone quality in bone strength and fracture risk is increasingly recognized. Finally, we can use preventive and therapeutical strategies, the efficacy of which has been unequivocally demonstrated in well-conducted randomized controlled trials, in women with postmenopausal osteoporosis, with fracture incidence as the primary end-point. In the long term, the devastating disabilities and other consequences of postmenopausal osteoporosis should be preventable. However, too many individuals, even with fragility fracture, are not investigated or treated adequately. It is therefore of utmost importance that a postmenopausal woman at risk of osteoporosis be identified and obtain adequate care. This is mandatory, otherwise the osteoporosis epidemic that is occuring as a consequence of increased life expectancy will impose on postmenopausal women a major threat to their quality of life and will be a major burden to the economy. Thus, our hope is that postmenopausal osteoporosis will become a disease of the past.

Index

adipocytic hormones 12
adipokines 11
adolescence see puberty
age factors 16, 26, 33, 38, 40, 43, 46, 58
alcohol intake 41
alendronate 61, 74, 78, 79, 87–88, 102, 103
amino acids 70–71
 see also protein
anabolic agents 65
androgens 16
anticatabolic agents 65
antiresorptive agents 69, 84–90
APD see pamidronate
axial compression 80

6-beta-catenin/Wnt-LRP5 signaling pathways 9
bisphosphonates 87–89, 101
BMC see bone mineral content
BMD see bone mineral density
body mass factors 19
bone mineral content (BMC) 18, 52, 53
bone mineral density (BMD) 3, 26, 29, 61, 66–67
 alendronate 103
 bisphosphonates 87, 103
 diagnoses 33, 35, 38–40, 43, 47, 49, 52–53, 55
 estrogen replacement therapy 27, 29
 exercise 95
 femoral neck bone 45
 hip fractures 47, 49
 lumbar spine 52
 mineral acquisition 17
 parathyroid hormone 91, 107
 proximal femur 53
 raloxifene 100
 risk factors 33
 strontium ranelate 93, 109
 tibolone 86
bones
 acquisition phases 3, 17–18
 anatomy/physiology 1–3
 cell development 2
 cell types 1
 composition 6
 dimensions 67–68
 formation phases 4, 9, 11, 13–14, 25–26, 62, 90–93, 110
 geometry 15, 61–62, 69
 histomorphometry 62, 73, 75
 loss 21–22, 24, 26, 29, 43
 macro/microarchitecture 1, 16, 62, 68, 71–72, 77
 mass 3, 12, 17, 19, 43, 67
 matrix/mineral composition 1, 6
 maximal loads 63, 69, 81
 mineralization 13
 modeling/remodeling processes 2–3, 5, 11, 12, 14, 25, 28, 63, 79
 peak bone mass 3, 17
 quality 61–82
 remodeling processes 5, 12, 25
 resorption phases 4, 11, 14, 25–26, 67, 84–90, 110
 size 68
 strength 61–82
broadband ultrasound attenuation (BUA) 54

C-terminal regions 91
calciotropic hormones 11
calcitonin 89, 106
calcitriol 29
calcium 17, 84
 early bone loss 29
 estrogen replacement 29
 institutionalized women 96
 nonpharmacological prevention/treatment 84, 94, 96
 pharmacological prevention/treatment 84–86, 111
 strontium ranelate 111
 young children 19

cancellous bone see trabecular bone
central nervous system (CNS) 12
chondrocytes 16
cigarette smoking 41, 84
CNS see central nervous system
collagen 1, 6
Colle's fracture 34, 49
common osteoporosis see idiopathic osteoporosis
compact bone see cortical bone
compression 46, 63, 80–81
computed tomography 36, 55, 62, 75–76
coregulator proteins 99
coronal magnetic resonance spin echo 57
cortical bone 1, 7, 21–22, 79, 80
coupling ultrasound media 54
cross-struts 77
CT scanners 76
CTX biochemical marker 40
cytokines 11, 23

denosumab 89–90
diagnoses 33–60
diet see nutrition
drugs 33, 83–114
'dry' ultrasound devices 54
dual-X-ray absorptiometry (DXA) 35–36, 51, 52, 53, 55
dynamic bone histomorphometric analyses 75

EC see external cortex
electronic digitizing 51
epidemiology 33–60
essential amino acids 70
estradiol 12, 99
estrogen
 bone microstructure 16
 deficiencies 4, 23–24, 26, 86
 receptor modulators 86–87, 99
 replacement therapy 27, 29, 86
 see also hormone replacement therapy
exercise 18, 83, 94–95
external cortex (EC) 15

fall prevention/protection 84, 94, 97
femoral neck bone 45, 48
 alendronate 103
 parathyroid hormone 107
 raloxifene 100
 strontium ranelate 92–93, 109
femur, proximal 53
FIT see Fracture Intervention Trial
FLEX see Fracture Intervention Trial Long-term Extension trial
fluoride treatment 61
forearm fractures 34
formation phases 9, 11, 25–26
 bone quality/strength 62
 estrogen deficiencies 4
 mineralization 13
 pharmacological prevention/treatment 90–93
 remodeling processes 14
 strontium ranelate 110
Fracture Intervention Trial (FIT) 102
Fracture Intervention Trial Long-term Extension (FLEX) trial 93
Fracture REduction Evaluation of Denosumab in Osteoporosis every 6 Months (FREEDOM) 89–90
Fracture Risk Assessment Tool (FRAX) 45
fractures
 age-related 38, 40, 43
 alcohol intake 41
 alendronate 102
 bisphosphonates 87–88
 calcitonin 106
 cigarette smoking 41
 diagnoses 33–60

economic costs 37, 57
 Genant's semiquantitative grading scale 56
 ibandronate 105
 independence/mortality/quality of life 37
 institutionalized women 96
 intervention goals 83
 Kaplan–Meier estimates 98
 mortality rates 58–59
 parathyroid hormone 90, 108
 pharmacological prevention/treatment 84–85
 prior/subsequent relationships 44
 raloxifene 100
 risedronate 104
 risk determinants 65
 sequelae 58
 strontium ranelate 111
 T-scores 42
 World Health Organization 45
 see also femoral neck bone; hip bone; vertebrae; wrist bone
fragility fractures 108
FRAX see Fracture Risk Assessment Tool
FREEDOM see Fracture REduction Evaluation of Denosumab in Osteoporosis every 6 Months

G-protein-coupled receptors 106
GCs see glucocorticoids
Genant's semiquantitative grading scale 56
genetic factors 3, 19, 20
genome wide association studies (GWAS) 20
GH see growth hormone
glucocorticoids (GCs) 5, 28
gonadal steroids see sex steroids
growth hormone (GH) 5, 12
GWAS see genome wide association studies

Haversian canal 22
high resolution peripheral quantitative computed tomography (HR-pQCT) 76
HIP see Hip Intervention Program study
hip bones 34, 39–40, 44, 47–49, 67
 alendronate 103
 bisphosphonates 87–89
 parathyroid hormone 107
 protection 94, 97
 risedronate 104
 strontium ranelate 91–92, 93, 109, 111
Hip Intervention Program (HIP) study 104
history-based diagnoses 34–35
hormone replacement therapy (HRT) 27, 29, 86, 98
HR-pQCT see high resolution peripheral quantitative computed tomography
humerus, proximal, 50

ibandronate 88, 105
idiopathic osteoporosis 20
IGF-1 see insulin-like growth factor-1
independent living 37
inhibitor cells 11
inorganic phases of bone composition 6
insulin-like growth factor-1 (IGF-1) 69
intertrochanteric fractures 48
isocaloric essential amino acid supplements 70
Kaplan–Meier estimates 98

leptin hormone 12
load–deflection curves 63, 81
lumbar spine see vertebrae

macrophage colony-stimulating factor (M-CSF) 8
markers 4, 25–26, 40, 63
maximal loads 63, 69, 81
menarcheal age 16
microcomputed tomography (microCT) 62, 75–76
microcracks 74

mineralization 13, 17–18, 63, 78
modeling processes 2–3
MORE see Multiple Outcomes of Raloxifene Evaluation trial
mortality 39, 58–59
Multiple Outcomes of Raloxifene Evaluation (MORE) trial
    100–101
mutations 3

nanoindentation studies 63, 71, 80
nitrogen-containing bisphosphonates 87, 101
non-nitrogen-containing bisphosphonates 101
noncollagenous proteins 1, 6
nonpharmacological prevention/treatment 83–84, 94–97
nutrition 5, 29, 84
    bone quality/strength 70
    calcium 19, 29–30, 84–86, 94, 96, 111
    protein 30, 70–71, 84
    vitamin D 5, 30, 84–86, 94, 96, 111
    young children 19

OBs see osteoblasts
OCs see osteoclasts
ONJ see osteonecrosis of the jaw
OPG see osteoprotegerin
organic phases of bone composition 6
osteoblasts (OBs) 1
    accelerated bone loss 22
    bone formation 9
    cell development 2
    estrogen deficiencies 4
    remodeling processes 14
    strontium ranelate 91, 110
    transcription factors 10
osteoclasts (OCs) 1
    accelerated bone loss 22
    cell development 2
    cross-section diagram 7
    differentiation 8
    estrogen deficiencies 4, 23
    remodeling processes 14
    strontium ranelate 91, 110
osteocytes 1, 4, 10, 22
osteonecrosis of the jaw (ONJ) 88–89
osteopenia 35, 46, 50–51, 55, 92–93
osteoporosis
    bone quality/strength 61–82
    definition 4
    epidemiology/diagnosis 33–60
    pathophysiology 1–33
    prevention/treatment 83–114
osteoprotegerin (OPG) 2, 91
ovariectomies 62, 66, 69
    amino acids 70
    mineralization 78
    pamidronate/parathyroid hormone 72
    remodeling processes 79

pamidronate (APD) 69, 72
parathyroid hormone (PTH) 106
    bone mass 12
    bone mineral density 107
    bone quality/strength 72
    nonvertebral fractures 108
    nutrition 29
    peptides 90–91
    pharmacological prevention/treatment 84–85
    remodeling processes 5, 12
    vertebral fractures 108

peak bone mass 3, 17
peptides 90–91
    see also protein
pharmacological prevention/treatment 84–93, 99–111
physical activity see exercise
physical examinations 34–35
polymorphisms 20
Prevent Recurrence of Osteoporotic Fractures (PROOF) 106
preventative measures 83–114
primary mineralization 13
protein 30, 70–71, 84, 99
PTH see parathyroid hormone
puberty 15, 17
pyrophosphate 101

quality of life 37
quantitative diagnoses 36, 37, 51, 54, 55, 56
quantitative microcomputed tomography
    see microcomputed tomography
quiescence phases 14

racial factors 34, 46
radiography
    alendronate/compact bone 79
    femoral neck bone 48
    hip fractures 48
    lumbar fractures 46
    osteopenia 50
    proximal humerus fractures 50
    vertebral fractures 36–37, 46
    wrist fractures 49
raloxifene 61, 99–100
receptor activator of nuclear factor kappa B ligand (RANKL)
    2, 8, 24, 91
remodeling processes 2–3, 5, 11–12, 14, 25, 28, 63, 79
resorption phases 11, 25–26
    antiresorptive agents 84–90
    bone quality/strength 67
    estrogen deficiencies 4
    remodeling processes 14
    strontium ranelate 110
reversal phases 14
risedronate 74, 87–88, 104
risk factors 33–34, 38–42
    alcohol intake 41
    alendronate 102
    bone quality/strength 65, 67
    cigarette smoking 41
    genetics 20
    hip fractures 67
    nonpharmacological prevention/treatment 94
    pharmacological prevention/treatment 84–85
    strontium ranelate 111
    T-scores 42
    World Health Organization 45

scintigraphy scans 37
secondary mineralization 13
selective estrogen receptor modulators (SERMs) 86–87, 99
semiquantitative (SQ) diagnoses 36–37, 56
sequelae 58
SERMs see selective estrogen receptor modulators
sex factors 58, 59
sex steroids 3, 12, 19, 62
    see also estrogen
sideways falls 97
single nucleotide polymorphisms (SNPs) 3, 20
Smith's fracture 34

smoking 41, 84
SNPs see single nucleotide polymorphisms
SOS see speed of sound
SOTI see Spinal Osteoporosis Therapeutic Intervention
    study
speed of sound (SOS) 54
Spinal Osteoporosis Therapeutic Intervention (SOTI) study
    91–93, 111
SQ see semiquantitative diagnoses
stimulator cells 11, 62
strontium ranelate 74, 91–93, 110
    bone mineral density 109
    hip fractures 111
    vertebral fractures 111
strontium ranelate treatment 81
subtrochanteric fractures 48

T-scores 35, 36, 38, 42
teriparatide 90–91
testosterone 12
TFs see transcription factors
thoracic vertebrae 57
three-point bending tests 63, 80
tibia, proximal 74
tibolone 86
tomography 36, 55, 62, 75–76
trabecular bone 1, 7, 21–22, 50, 80
transcription factors (TFs) 2, 10
transiliac bone biopsies 75
TReatment Of Peripheral OSteoporosis (TROPOS) 91–93, 111
treatments 83–114
turnover see remodeling processes

ultrasound 36, 54, 55

vertebrae 34, 44, 46, 52
    alendronate 103
    amino acids 70
    bone mineral density 52
    bone quality/strength 64
    calcitonin 106
    compression tests 81
    coronal magnetic resonance spin echo 57
    Genant's semiquantitative grading scale 56
    ibandronate 88, 105
    parathyroid hormone 90, 107, 108
    radiological assessments 36–37
    raloxifene 100
    risedronate 104
    strontium ranelate 91–93, 109
vertebral body quantitative morphometry 51
vitamin D 5, 30, 84
    institutionalized women 96
    nonpharmacological prevention/treatment 84, 94, 96
    pharmacological prevention/treatment 84–86, 111
    strontium ranelate 111

'wet' ultrasound devices 54
Wnt-LRP5/6-beta-catenin signaling pathways 9
Women's Health Initiative (WHI) 86, 98
World Health Organization (WHO) 45, 51
wrist bone 44, 49

X-ray absorptiometry 35–36, 51, 52, 53, 55
Xtreme CT scanners 76

Z-scores 35, 36
zoledronic acid 88

Index compiled by Indexing Specialists (UK) Ltd, www.indexing.co.uk, phone +44 (0)1273 416 777.